A QUIVER BOOK

THE SEX BIBLE

FOR PEOPLE OVER 50

*The Complete Guide to Sexual Love
for Mature Couples*

LAURIE BETITO, PH.D.

The Sex Bible for People Over Fifty

Text © 2014 Fair Winds Press/Quiver
Photography © 2014 Fair Winds Press/Quiver

First published in the USA in 2014 by
Fair Winds Press/Quiver, a member of
Quarto Publishing Group USA Inc.
100 Cummings Center
Suite 406-L
Beverly, MA 01915-6101
www.fairwindspress.com
Visit http://bodymindbeautyhealth.com.
It's your personal guide to a happy, healthy,
and extraordinary life!

All rights reserved. No part of this book
may be reproduced or utilized, in any form
or by any means, electronic or mechanical,
without prior permission in writing from the
publisher.

17 16 15 14   1 2 3 4 5

ISBN: 978-1-59233-500-8

Digital edition published in 2014
eISBN: 978-1-62788-043-5

Library of Congress Cataloging-in-
Publication Data available

Cover and book design by Burge Agency
Photography by Ed Fox, edfox.com
Makeup and hair by Kelly Oleary
Photo retouching by Alex C Retouch
Photos on pages 49, 57, 107, 130, 132, 133,
and 134 courtesy of Lucia Scarlotta.

Printed and bound in Hong Kong

The information in this book is for
educational purposes only. It is not intended
to replace the advice of a physician or
medical practitioner. Please see your health
care provider before beginning any new
health program.

TO JOEL, MY LOVING,
WONDERFUL HUSBAND OF
20 YEARS . . . THE BEST YEARS
ARE AHEAD OF US!

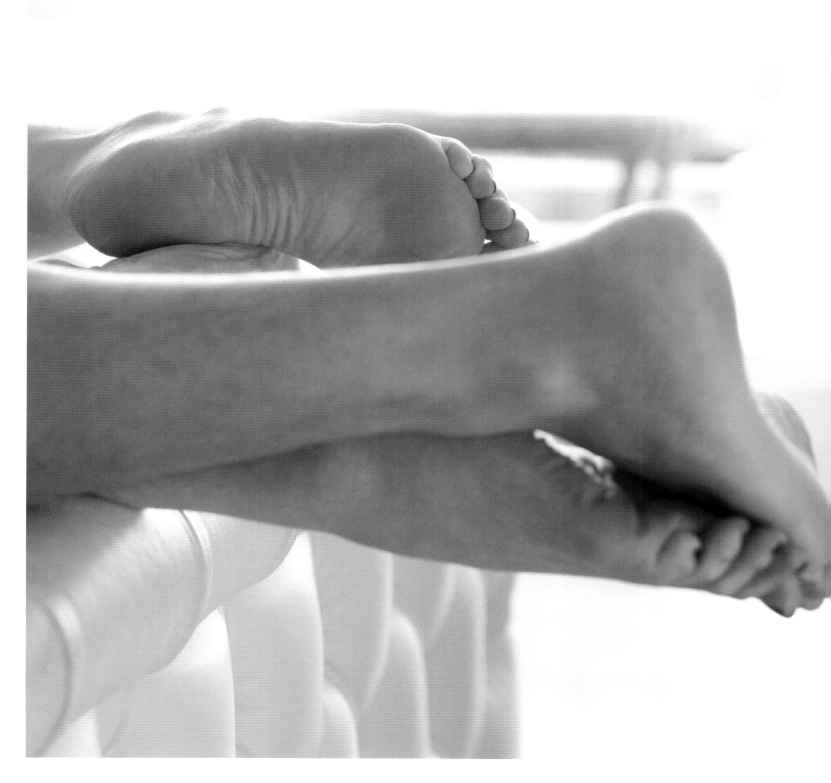

Contents

Foreword

Until sixteen years ago, doctors, sex researchers, and sex therapists didn't know very much about mature people's sexuality. But in 1998, the approval of Viagra triggered an explosion of research into lovemaking after fifty, and today we know more about later-life sex than ever before.

For instance, intercourse fades from the repertoire. Even with erection medication, some mature men don't have erections sufficiently firm for intercourse. And despite lubricants, vaginal dryness and atrophy may make intercourse uncomfortable or impossible for many older women. However, there are plenty of ways to enjoy marvelous, intimate, deeply satisfying sex that don't involve intercourse. Surveys agree that with the right attitude and a few adjustments, no one is too old for sex, no matter how long they live.

Which brings me to the marvelous book you hold in your hands. Laurie Betito, Ph.D., is a prominent, very experienced, and highly regarded sex therapist, and her book combines vast clinical experience with wonderful insights into the latest research on sex after fifty. She dispels the many myths that still haunt our culture and declares that sex after fifty can be the best sex of your life. That assertion is no exaggeration. It's based on the findings of a huge body of research by scientists all over the world.

Dr. Betito describes:
• How sex enhances mature lovers' physical and mental health and even extends longevity.
• Why menopause does not mean the end of satisfying sex for women. With the right attitude and a few adjustments, menopause can actually herald an erotic renaissance.
• Why mature men's iffy erections and even erectile dysfunction do not mean the end of enjoyable sex.
• How libido evolves in later adulthood, and how to keep the erotic fires burning.

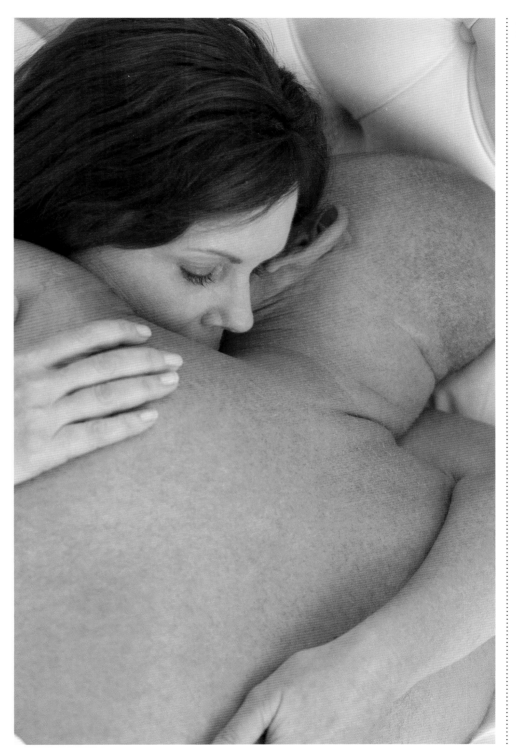

• How to set the mood for lovemaking after fifty.
• How mature lovers can continue to enjoy intercourse if they can manage it, and, if not, how they can have deeply satisfying sex without it.
• How age-related health concerns affect sex and how to enjoy lovemaking despite them.
• How some new erotic tricks can be great boons to mature lovers.

So forget everything you've ever heard about sexuality supposedly peaking at eighteen or twenty-five or thirty, and going downhill from there. Lovemaking and the intimacy that both fuels and deepens it are gifts that last a lifetime. Despite the physical challenges of growing older, you can enjoy marvelous sex at any age. *The Sex Bible for People Over Fifty* shows you how.

Michael Castleman
Author of *Great Sex: A Man's Guide to the Secrets of Total-Body Lovemaking*, publisher of www.GreatSexAfter40.com, and writer of the blog *All About Sex* for www.PsychologyToday.com

Introduction

Whenever I attend a dinner party, people inevitably begin telling me about their sex lives within minutes of discovering that I'm a sex therapist. And the most frequent question I get (bearing in mind that the parties I go to are usually attended by couples between the ages of forty and sixty) is some variation of "How can I spice up my marriage and get my drive back?"

What I tell them: The very first thing they need to understand is that, as we age, our bodies change, and with these changes comes the need to adapt. This means that we must adjust our expectations and be open to learning new things. We need a different sexual skill set in our fifties and sixties than we had in our twenties and thirties.

Reality check: Sex at sixty-five won't be the same as it was at twenty-five, but that doesn't mean it can't be great, even the best ever. This is a time of life when we can feel more free— free of pregnancy fears, free of little ones barging into the bedroom, free to take more time for ourselves. It's vital that you learn to go with the flow of your changing body—and take charge of what you can do to make yourself feel good.

I'm a clinical psychologist with a specialty in sex therapy. I have been seeing clients for the past twenty-five years. Much of what I do involves helping couples (and singles) achieve their full sexual potential. I've also dedicated much of my career to sex education. My nightly radio show provides me the perfect opportunity to reach tens of thousands of people—what a privilege!

My goals have always been to start the conversation about sex, bring it out of the closet and into the open, and let people know that they are not alone (or "abnormal"). So, why a book about sex specifically for couples over fifty? I needed to write this book for several reasons. One was selfish: Turning fifty, and having a husband over fifty, I wanted to make sure I had explored every avenue to ensure that we continue to have great sex. Second, much of my work with couples over fifty involves answering questions about what is "normal" sex and helping them deal with the sexual changes that age has brought about. Third, most of my listeners are over the age of forty, and the questions I get from them often have to do with such changes. They seek my reassurance that what they are experiencing is in fact "normal for my age."

I felt that an open discussion about sex and aging was necessary, and I wanted to reach an even wider audience. My whole career has been about having frank, open, uncensored discussions about a topic that's not always easy to confront. Over the years, I've probably fielded thousands of questions about sex on the air. One thing I've learned, and what I tell my listeners, is that if one caller is asking a question, then you can bet one hundred listeners have asked themselves the exact same one.

Let's head back to that dinner party. The *second* most frequent question I get from couples over fifty is "Why are we having sex so much less than everyone else?" I'm going to tell you what I tell them, usually to their great relief: The general public, no matter the age, is *not* having sex every morning, afternoon, and evening, in every room of the house, switching to a new position every thirty seconds!

Sure, a study from the University of Colorado in Boulder recently concluded that having regular sex makes people a little happier. But there's a catch: Our happiness hinges not just on how much sex we're having, but also on how often we have sex *in comparison to how often we believe our peers are doing it*. What makes us happy, it seems, is knowing that we measure up—that we are "normal."

Yet we're bombarded with stories in the media that would have us believe that we're sexually dysfunctional or aberrant. An often-quoted study (Laumann and colleagues, 1999) estimated that almost half of American women suffer from some form of sexual dysfunction—namely, low sexual desire. *Half the population?* Wouldn't that then make low sexual desire the norm? Are half of us really dysfunctional just because we don't always feel like having sex, or do we merely express our sexuality differently?

That's not to say that some of us don't experience dysfunction. As a point of reference, for a sexual issue to qualify as a dysfunction—for it to be a problem—you have to be distressed by it. No distress, no dysfunction . . . merely a variation.

In fact, according to the National Bureau of Economic Research, the average American has sex two or three times a month. For people over the age of forty, that number is once a month. If you really want to know how often the average middle-aged couple has sex, you'll have to ask them. If you and your partner have sex twice per week, then your average is twice per week. The only time the frequency becomes problematic is when one partner isn't on the same page as the other. I'll explore that issue in depth in chapter 5.

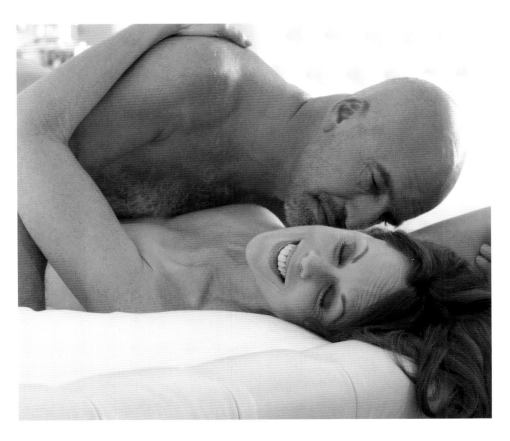

AM I "DYSFUNCTIONAL"?

Before labeling yourself sexually dysfunctional*, ask yourself these three questions:

Does my sexual situation cause me marked distress?

Does my sexual situation cause me any interpersonal difficulties?

Is my sexual situation a result of a medical condition or medication?

If you answered "Yes," "Yes," and No," then you should get a thorough sexological evaluation. To find a sex therapist near you, visit www.aasect.org or www.aamft.org.

* According to the *Diagnostic and Statistical Manual of Mental Disorders* (*DSM-5*)

IS THIS BOOK FOR YOU?

This book is for you, a couple in your late forties, fifties, or early sixties (and beyond) who are still attracted to each other and who want to "get it back." You had an active sex life once, you enjoy sex, you may or may not have experimented with some boundaries, and you know what you like. Maybe you're a little set in your ways. Now, you want more.

This book is for you if you're going through the typical physical changes that aging bodies succumb to—aches and pains, the effects of menopause or erectile difficulties—or going through the emotional changes that may accompany you as you journey through your life. Whether you're experiencing fear of abandonment as you start over and seek companionship, dealing with a new sense of identity (as parents or grandparents instead of a sexual heartthrob), noticing hormonal changes, or discovering new societal norms (such as the acceptance of online dating), things aren't the same as they used to be.

This book is for you if want to continue to be as sexually active as when you were younger, but struggle to calibrate to the changes that have been forced upon you by time.

This book is for you if you want answers and results *now*. You want a how-to manual for getting back to great sex and a guide who understands your needs and what you go through as a person of a certain age, including the relationship challenges you may be having. You want to learn new skills, new positions, and new techniques.

Some of the topics I'll cover in the following pages are:
• *Surprising truths about sex and aging.* Recent findings show that many common myths about sexuality—such as "libido declines," "the quality of sex diminishes," or "erectile dysfunction is inevitable" with age—are just that: myths. This book will show you the facts and help put the myths into perspective.
• *The health benefits of sex for aging adults.* Why have sex at all? What's in it for you? Pure pleasure, emotionally healthier intimacy, and a physically healthier you are a few. What better reasons do you need?
• *How aging affects men's and women's sexuality.* Aging is inevitable, and priorities do change, but our emotional needs and our sexual brains are still as young as ever.
• *How to rekindle desire.* Together we'll explore techniques and strategies to reawaken the passion in you.
• *Specific tips and techniques for intercourse, non-penetrative sex, and "spicier" sex.* Sex doesn't begin and end with the missionary position. I hope this book will incite you to try new positions and techniques to enhance your sex life.

If you want more and better sex, then this book is for you.

GET READY
FOR A GREAT
SEX LIFE

I want this book to be your bedside companion, offering you concrete tips and advice. Each chapter will discuss a specific aspect of sexuality and give you exercises, tips, and techniques you can try. It will teach you what you can do to ignite desire, spice things up with your partner, and make sex thoroughly enjoyable. I want you to celebrate sexuality.

What's important is to take charge of your sexuality. Prioritize fun and pleasure—including sexual pleasure. In this book, I'm going to show you how to do exactly that. Sex can and should be fun, and it can also help keep us young physically, mentally, and emotionally. It's time for the post-fifty crowd to let go of the notion that they have to compete with their younger counterparts. Experience, enthusiasm, and maturity are all sexy.

The bottom line: Great sex can be yours for many, many years to come. Welcome to the next stage of your sex life!

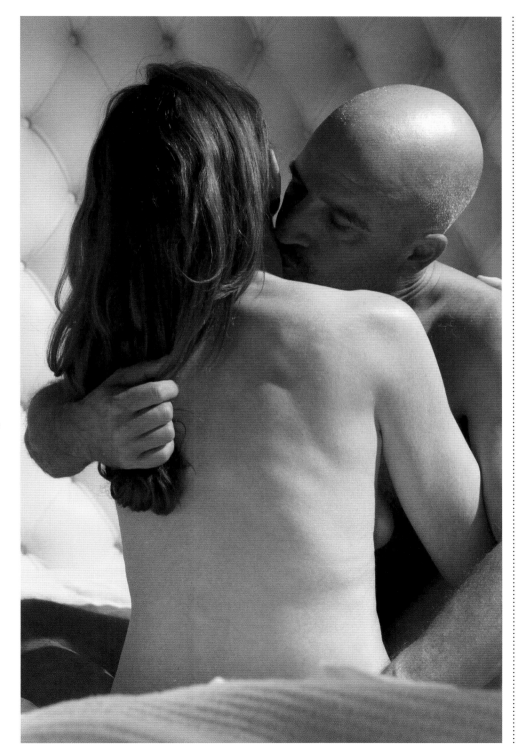

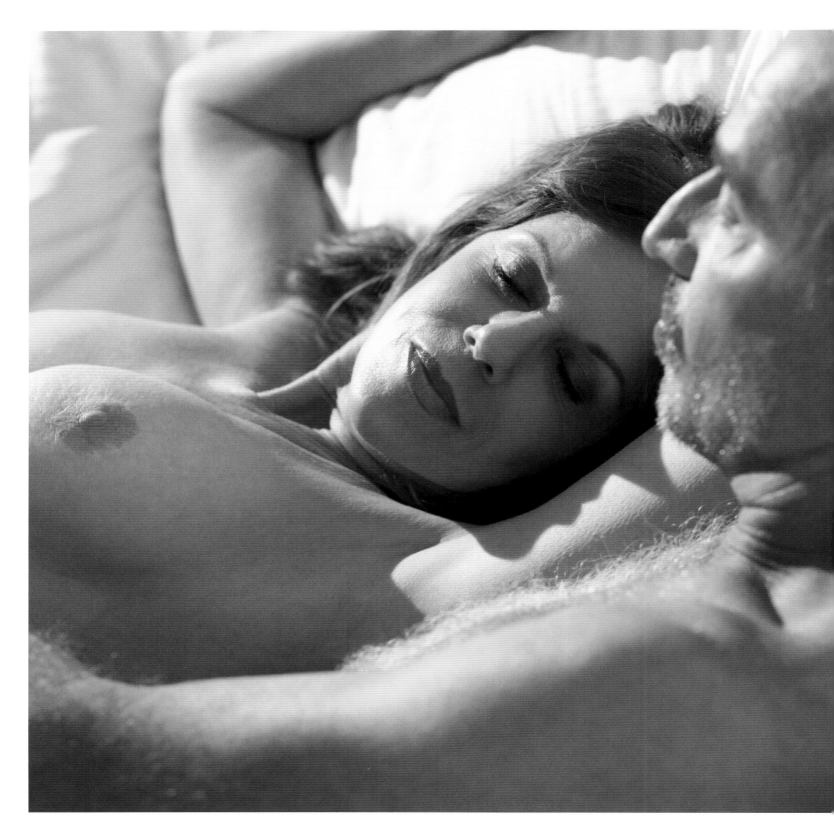

⚥01

Sex Doesn't Have an Expiration Date!

Sexuality is a gift that we can keep well into our eighties, and if we're lucky, even beyond. Unfortunately, it's a gift that's too often associated with youth, especially in Western cultures. And some people come to experience sex as a burden or chore—it becomes just one more thing they have to do for their partner. But does the march of time mean you have to give up on one of life's gifts? NO! This book will help. But before you find your frisky again, discover what you need and learn how to ask for it, and follow your path to greater sexual pleasure, let's look at some of the misconceptions around aging and sex.

RESPECTED ELDER OR OLD WOMAN?

In some Asian cultures, women experience menopause as a rite of passage that marks them as having a higher status—one of Respected Elder. They are seen as free from the duties of motherhood and worries about unwanted reproduction. In contrast, Western women often view this transition as bringing a loss of societal status. Menopause is perceived as the point at which a woman has entered old age. Sadly, it's also often viewed as the end of sexuality.

How a woman responds to menopause may depend partly on external factors such as culture. But it's her *attitude* that will trump everything and determine whether she feels empowered.

FIVE MYTHS ABOUT SEX AFTER FIFTY

In our society, we hold on to many myths about aging. What lies behind them is our fear of growing old, embarrassment and discomfort around sexuality, misinformation and outdated information, and of course, the cultural idealization of youth. Here are some of the most common myths about sex after fifty—followed by the realities.

MYTH #1: SEXUALLY, WOMEN PEAK IN THEIR THIRTIES.

Fact: Hormonally, both men *and* women peak somewhere around age eighteen, when they're considered at the height of their sexual functioning. Of course, a "peak" implies a decline afterward, and although it's true that hormone levels begin to drop very slowly after eighteen, most people barely notice it. In fact, according to the Sinclair Intimacy Institute, and through my own conversations, many women report the best sex of their lives much later in life and say that their capacity for orgasm doesn't diminish with age. They say they're enjoying sex more because they're no longer worried about getting pregnant.

According to a survey commissioned by *Top Santé* magazine and reported by *The Telegraph* newspaper, married women over forty are having the best sex of their lives. More than 80 percent of those polled said they were more sexually adventurous now than when they were in their twenties, while 63 percent said that sex was better because they'd become more sexually confident over the years. In another survey conducted by *Saga Magazine* of nine thousand people over the age of fifty, one-third of the women who responded said sex is more enjoyable now than it was when they were in their youth.

These sentiments echo what marital and sex therapist David Schnarch, Ph.D., says in his book *Passionate Marriage: Keeping Love and Intimacy Alive in Committed Relationships*: "The speed with which your body responds is only one measure of sexual prime. Your sexual peak has a great deal to do with who you are as a person."

MYTH #2: THE ORGASMS YOU HAVE WHEN YOU'RE YOUNG ARE BETTER AND MORE INTENSE.

Fact: Many women report that their orgasms became more intense and more fulfilling after they turned forty. Several have even reported experiencing female ejaculation

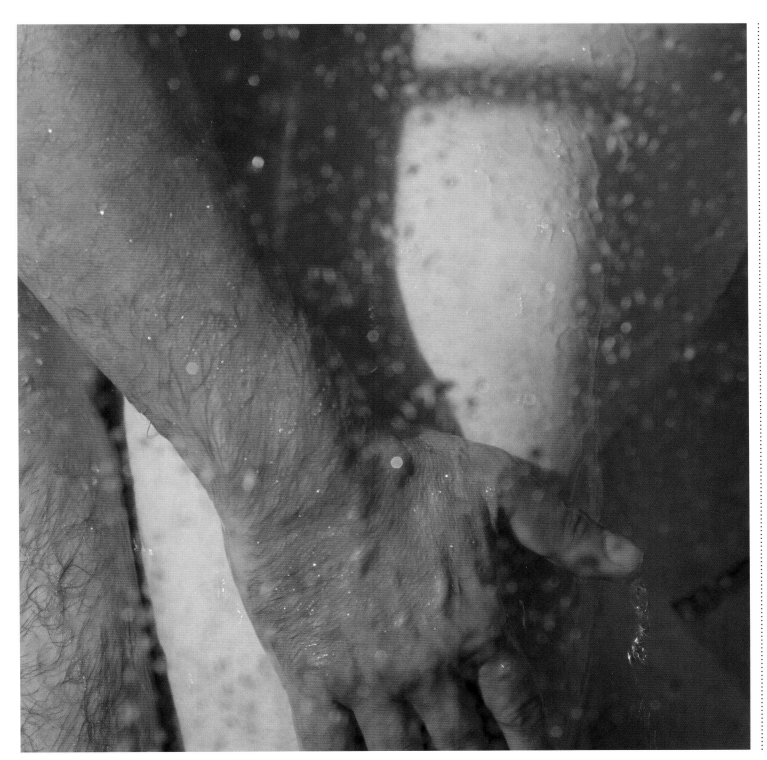

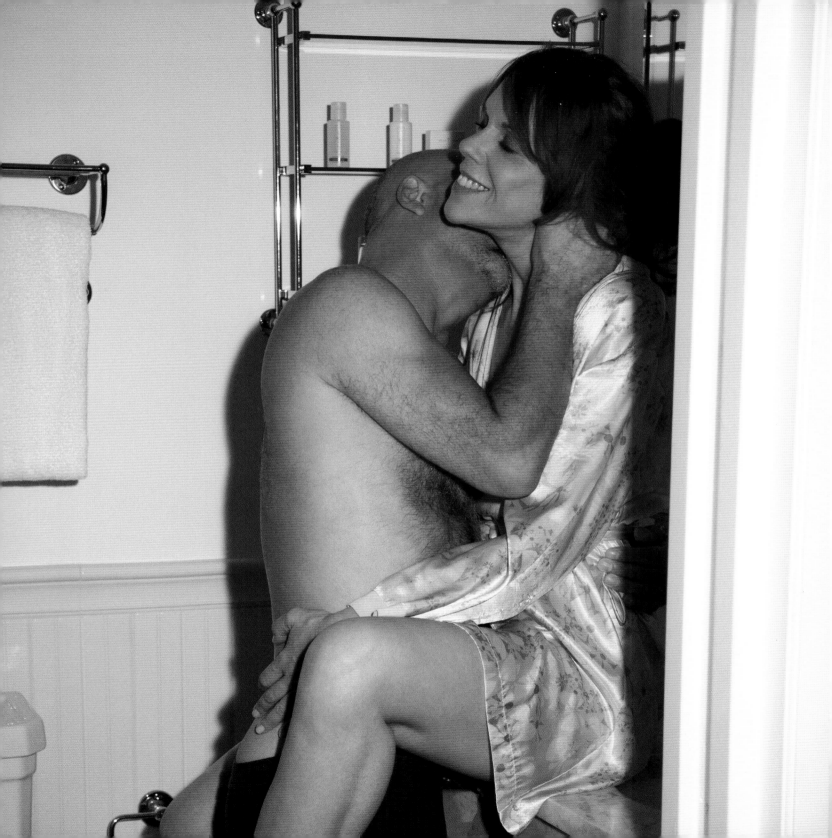

for the very first time! Mature women have a better understanding of what makes them tick sexually, and they are less afraid to ask for what they want. (I'll talk about ways to do this later in the book.) Author Joel Block, Ph.D., goes as far as saying, in his book *Secrets of Better Sex: A Noted Sex Therapist Reveals His Secrets to Passionate Sexual Fulfillment*, that women in midlife are more likely to have multiple orgasms than at any other time in their lives.

As for men, although it's true that the force of ejaculation gets weaker with age, many men experience a more diffuse, all-over-body orgasm that may be even more intense.

MYTH #3: ERECTION PROBLEMS ARE INEVITABLE.

Fact: Most men experience erectile dysfunction (ED) occasionally, and the majority of them will never need treatment. Over the years, however, I've seen countless men in an absolute panic because they thought they could no longer get an erection. If men could accept that their penises may sometimes "fail" them, and go on to enjoy

other forms of sexuality, then they would learn that they have other wonderful skills they can use to stimulate their partners. At such times, their partners are generally grateful not to be rushed into intercourse before the erection is gone. And so what if it is? Use it as an opportunity to try some of the "outercourse" techniques in chapter 8.

MYTH #4: WE LOSE INTEREST IN SEX AS WE GET OLDER.

Fact: Our spontaneous desire or "need" for it may wane, but our interest does not. If the *Fifty Shades of Grey* phenomenon is any indication, then interest in sex is alive and well. Many women of all ages passed around those books like they were an exciting discovery. They were full of new sexual thoughts, conversations, and activities.

But the way women and men experience sexual interest does differ. The work of sex researcher Rosemary Basson, M.D., on female desire beautifully explains how desire in women is not triggered in the same way as it is for men. For the most part, men

CASE STUDY: JANET

Janet, a fifty-two-year-old mother of teenagers, sought therapy because she felt she had "lost herself." She was having a difficult time enjoying life, including sex. We worked on strategies to cope with feelings of guilt and resentment, figuring out what she needed to do to feel better about herself. She started doing yoga, going to the gym, and meditating, which in turn made her calmer, more flexible, and more sexual. She and her husband started going out on "dates" more, even taking overnight mini-vacations together. Both reported a much more satisfying relationship.

are triggered by visual cues, and they seem more easily able to separate what goes on around them from their sexual feelings. Women, on the other hand, are much more contextual. What goes on around them often can greatly affect their interest in sex at any given time. As the old saying goes: Men can have sex in a pigsty, but for women, one sock on the floor can be enough to distract them from sex. Essentially, a woman may think about sex and want to have sex with her mate (in other words, *be interested* in sex), not necessarily because she's horny (spontaneous desire for sex), but because the context is just right.

Thus, if we take into account these differences, then we would see the distinction between desire and interest and not confound the two. It's a question of stimulating that interest to create the desire, which I discuss in chapter 5.

MYTH #5: THE QUALITY OF SEX DECLINES AS WE AGE.

Fact: The quality of sex actually improves with age as we gain confidence and knowledge. There's more focus on sensuality and foreplay, which makes sex even better. My mature clients regularly describe experiencing their orgasms throughout their bodies as opposed to only in their genitals. They describe sex as almost a spiritual experience.

Because there are so many myths about sex after fifty, it's that much more important to distinguish misinformation from fact. Educate yourself as much as possible about the new skill sets you need to enhance your sexual experience. These skills include:
• Developing a good attitude
• Communicating your desires (clearly and lovingly) to your partner
• Changing up your sexual routine
• Focusing on foreplay
• Exploring previously neglected body parts such as the perineum, anus, and prostate
• Exploring new positions
• Focusing on more direct genital stimulation through oral sex or the use of sex toys
• Learning to take care of your genitals to keep them in top working order

Sound like a tall order? It's not. I'll discuss these skills in detail in the next chapters.

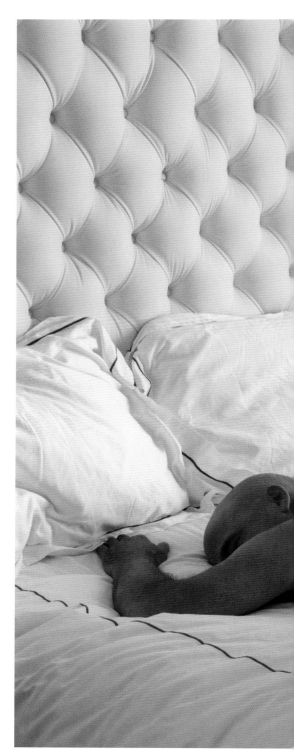

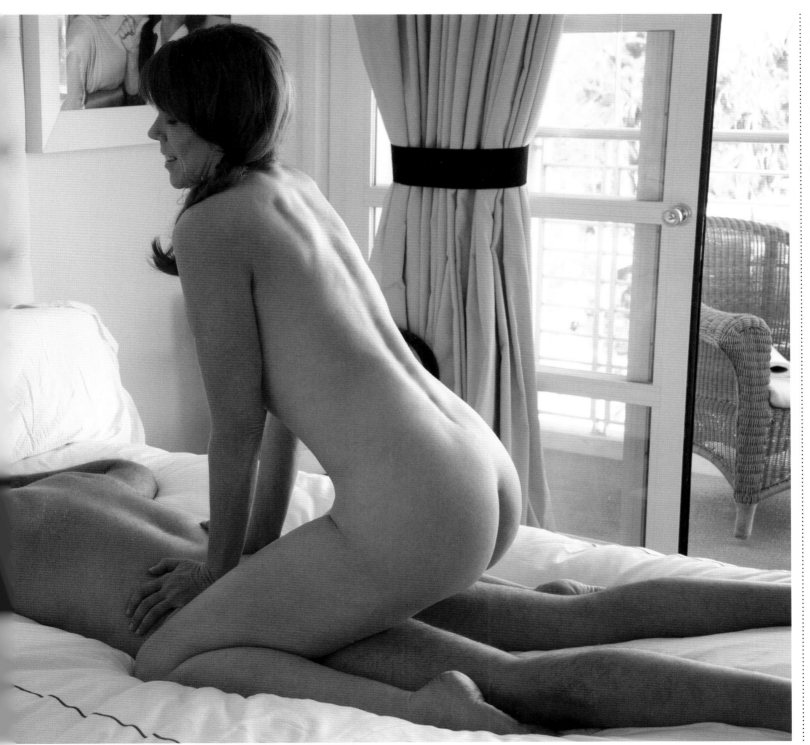

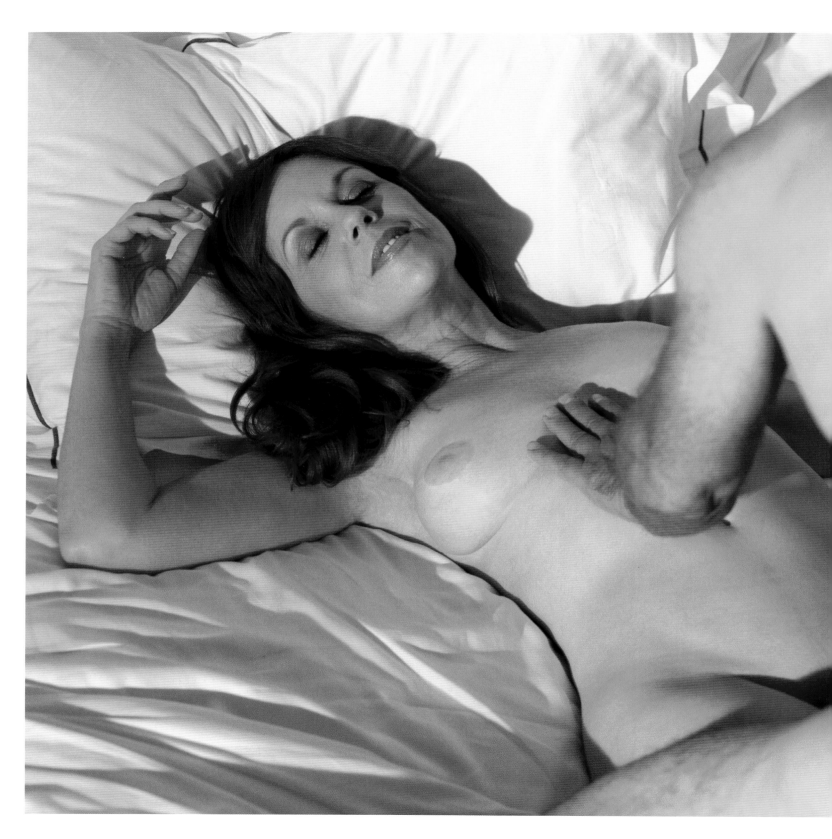

02

Why Have Sex? It's Good for You!

There's no getting around it: Our bodies change as we age. How *yours* changes depends on a number of factors—including your genes, diet, exercise routine, family environment, and ability to manage stress. If you've taken relatively good care of yourself, you may get compliments such as, "You look great for your age!" As backhanded compliments go, it's still much better than hearing the opposite. But there's a way to improve your life that's always been within your reach, regardless of your age: sex.

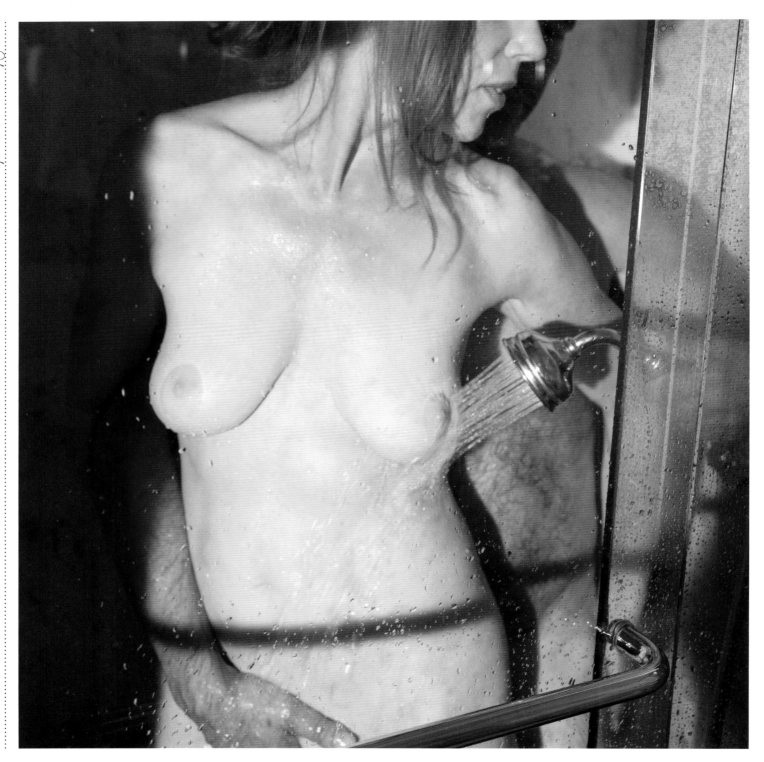

Jake and Susan, a couple in their late sixties, were having trouble because he was having difficulty maintaining an erection. The couple also had trouble discussing sex, so they just avoided it altogether. They were beginning to argue over little things. He became grumpy, and she was resentful because Jake was avoiding all forms of touch with her.

They were coached to start building some sexual intimacy by focusing first on nonsexual touching. Over the course of several months, they intensified the touch. Both reported feeling much closer and less resentful. Eventually, they resumed intercourse once Jake's physical issues were dealt with. As Susan said, "Now that we have sexual contact regularly—even if it's not intercourse—he's so much nicer! We hardly argue anymore."

THE BENEFITS OF BEING SEXUALLY ACTIVE PAST FIFTY

Regardless of the challenges your age brings, you have the ability to tap into the "miracle cure" that happens to be sex. Think of sex as a trunk full of magical elixirs, each one a little different from the next, but all able to captivate you and your partner under a spell of pleasure. All you have to do is find the right combination of sexual remedies to meet your needs and take your existing health and relational challenges into consideration.

Having a regular sex life, coupled or solo, can provide a multitude of health benefits, some of which can be used to enhance the moment, and others that will serve you well for the rest of your life.

There are many physical benefits to having regular sex, but if you're in a relationship, the advantages take on a more holistic theme in terms of the payback you receive mentally and emotionally. Lovemaking will connect you as a couple and build the intimacy level every time. Even if you've had a bad day with each other, the physical connection will help you overcome problems time and again. You'll inevitably feel desired and loved by your partner and, as a result, you'll feel sexier.

When a couple's sex life is unfulfilling, it usually ends up turning into a larger issue that can threaten the relationship. Conversely, if you're satisfied with your sex life, then sex is not THE most important factor in your relationship. Nor should it be. Sex should be a physical expression of the emotional attachment you feel. What follows are just a few of the many reasons why sex is oh-so-good for you—no matter what your age, but especially for those in the second half of their lives.

SEX HEALS

Mature adults can get too comfortable with chronic pain. Whether it's from an injury that never quite healed or a tolerance built up over time for prescription pain medication, pain is often accepted as part of daily life. That's why adults over fifty can more easily push off sex when the symptoms of a headache or other pain are on the attack. A person who's in the mood can be stopped cold when his or her significant other has throbbing temples.

But be mindful of just how easily "not tonight, dear" can then be invoked tomorrow night, the rest of the week, the rest of the month . . . and then one day you wake up and wonder how you went from a sexually active partner to a sexless and distant roommate. The paradox is that one of the best ways to resolve headache pain—or any kind of pain, in fact—is sex. Headaches are caused when the blood vessels in your head constrict. Sexual intercourse alleviates that tension and causes those blood vessels to expand, thus relieving your headache.

What's more, your body releases the hormone oxytocin when you're sexually aroused, creating a feeling of well-being and contentment, as well as positive feelings toward your partner. From a biological perspective, sex—as well as cuddling, kissing, and other sexual activities—breeds feelings of love and attachment. Oxytocin (the "love hormone") and other neurochemicals are released upon intimate touch and greatly increase feelings of love, trust, security, and bonding. In both men and women, oxytocin levels rise dramatically during orgasm. At the same time, the body releases the neurotransmitter dopamine, which creates a strong sense of pleasure, excitement, and well-being. The combined effects of oxytocin and dopamine cause you to associate your sexual partner with a sense of pleasure as well. And as a bonus, oxytocin contributes to reducing pain and even increases your threshold for migraines and other ailments.

In addition to oxytocin, other pain-relieving elements flood the body during sex. Professor Stuart Brody, Ph.D., in discussing his study published in the *Bulletin of Experimental Biology and Medicine*, says, "Sex boosts endorphins, the body's natural painkillers, by up to a third in a matter of minutes. There's evidence this helps a wide range of conditions, including lower-back pain, migraine, and arthritis. And although it's less reliable and effective than drug therapies, the pain-relieving effects of orgasm are quicker."

One side effect of the release of oxytocin during orgasm is that it helps you fall asleep (so if your partner falls asleep after sex, *it's a good thing*). Sex is the safest and most natural "over-the-counter" sleeping aid that exists.

SEX REDUCES STRESS

More experienced adults may not have the same challenges as those starting out with new families or careers, but that doesn't mean that their problems are any less stressful. Sex is a healthy option for coping with all kinds of stress.

Although you might not feel like making love after a bad commute or when you're worried about your 401(k) or I.R.A., sex can lower blood pressure and overall stress levels, regardless of age. It releases tension, elevates mood, and creates a profound sense of relaxation, especially in the postcoital period. From a biochemical perspective, sex causes the release of endorphins and increases levels of white blood cells that actually boost the immune system. Researchers have found that even non-penetrative sex—which can include simply hugging, touching, and kissing—can have this effect (see chapter 8). In fact, a study published in the journal *Biological Psychology* described how men who had had sex the previous night responded better to stressful situations! It makes sense: If you're regularly sexual, you're regularly relaxed, and when you're relaxed, you cope better with stressful situations. Life feels more positive.

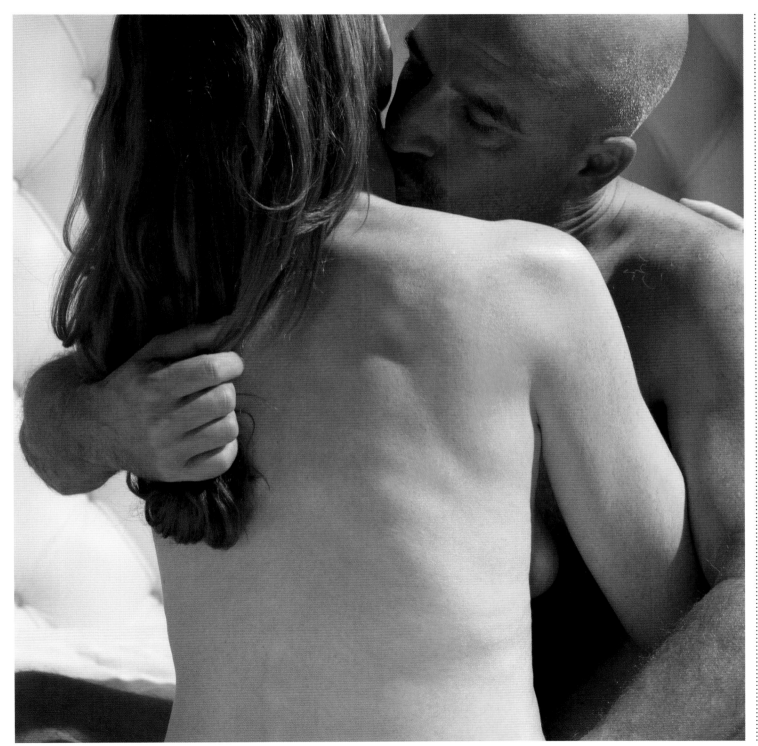

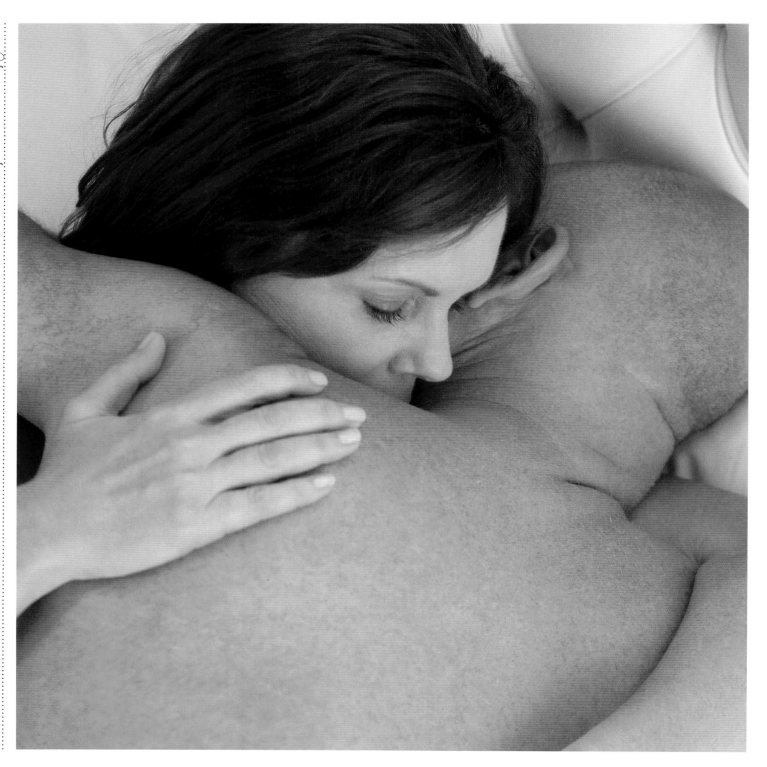

And sex is a gift that keeps on giving. A 2007 study published in the *Archives of Sexual Behavior* reported that sexual behavior with a partner on one day significantly predicted lower negative mood and stress, and higher positive mood, on the following day.

SEX INCREASES OVERALL HAPPINESS

Although every stage of life brings challenges with it, if you're over fifty, you're probably juggling a specific set of issues. You may still be parenting children or teenagers— or conversely, dealing with empty-nest syndrome. You might be a caregiver for aging parents while trying to manage your own medical issues. Having regular sex can help you approach these challenges with a more positive attitude. Sex can:

• Give people a more positive outlook on life.
• Diminish feelings of insecurity by making people feel sexy, vibrant, and desirable.
• Increase self-esteem—very few people are capable of feeling terrible about themselves while having an orgasm!
• Reconfirm levels of commitment and keep partners more connected.
• Encourage a more youthful attitude.

SEX IMPROVES FITNESS AND OVERALL HEALTH

A large survey published in the *New England Journal of Medicine* of more than three thousand participants aged fifty-seven to eighty-five found that those who were having regular sex rated their general health higher than those who weren't. Regular sexual activity improves memory, reduces cholesterol levels, increases circulation, and raises energy levels. It also burns up to 250 calories every half hour. Those minutes add up! And the more you have sex, the more stamina you'll have, so you'll be able to last longer. It's just like when you go to the gym regularly—you feel energized and confident, your self-esteem is higher, and you have better focus. Simply put, you feel better.

Sex has specific benefits for each gender. For men, one of the more apparent physical benefits is a healthier prostate. A study of 30,000 men by Michael Leitzmann, M.D., Ph.D., M.P.H., while a researcher at the National Cancer Institute in Bethesda, Maryland, found that men who enjoy an active sex life have a reduced risk of prostate cancer in later life. His findings indicated that men who ejaculate between thirteen and twenty times a month had a 14 percent lower risk of prostate cancer than men who ejaculated between four and seven times a month. Men who ejaculated more than twenty-one times a month had a 33 percent lower lifetime risk of prostate cancer. The researchers believe that sexual activity has a protective effect because the prostate secretes the bulk of the fluid in semen, and climaxing may flush out cancer-causing agents. Another possible explanation is that ejaculation reduces the development of calcifications that have been linked to cancer.

Meanwhile, the Duke Study on Aging found that the more a woman enjoys sex, the longer her life span. Women who have regular sex maintain healthier vaginas, because sexual activity increases blood flow, which nourishes the vaginal walls, resulting in a moister, more elastic vagina. This happens because sexual activity helps regulate estrogen levels and promotes greater estrogen production. It's the estrogen that maintains an optimal vaginal environment— which, in turn, is better for intercourse. Don't have a partner? You can keep your vagina healthy by using sex toys.

ONE WOMAN'S ANSWER

At a talk I was giving about how to keep passion alive, a woman, around the age of forty shared a story that had all the other women falling off their chairs. She described how every night before she goes to bed she performs oral sex on her husband. She said that while she feels neutral about the act itself, it only took about two minutes of her time, and she reaped the benefits every day. "When my husband gets his sex regularly, he's an absolute pussy cat, and I get to do what I want, when I want!" she said. She started using this strategy after she saw how crabby he was when she kept refusing to have sex. The women in the room were appalled that this woman was "giving" her husband so much sex. She set them straight, saying that she was doing it for herself. She felt like she gained more than he did! For this couple, the approach worked.

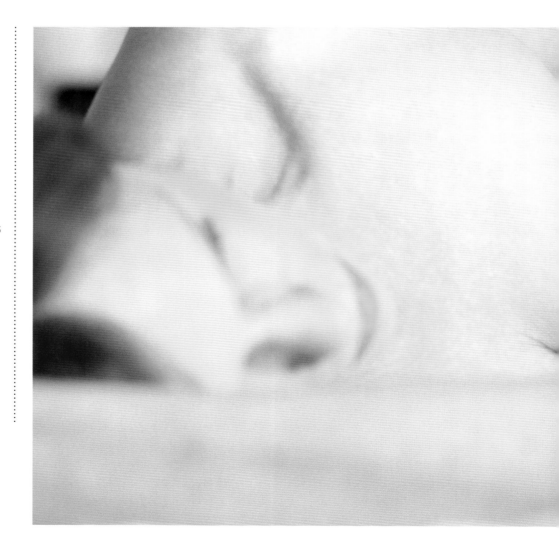

SEX SLOWS AGING

Another benefit of sex can be seen immediately after orgasm, when we're basking in the afterglow and our faces are flushed from the increase in blood flow. David Weeks, M.D., while at the Royal Edinburgh Hospital in Scotland, conducted a study of 3,500 people between the ages of 18 and 105. Volunteer judges found that the couples who were having sex at least three times per week looked on average *seven to twelve years younger* than their counterparts who were having less sex! Apparently, sex helps boost the skin's production of vitamin D and estrogen, which can make your skin smoother and your hair shinier. Weeks commented: "Sex triggers human growth hormone, which combats free radicals from pollution and exposure to other damaging environmental factors. This helps preserve skin cell walls and relax muscles that could otherwise cause wrinkles."

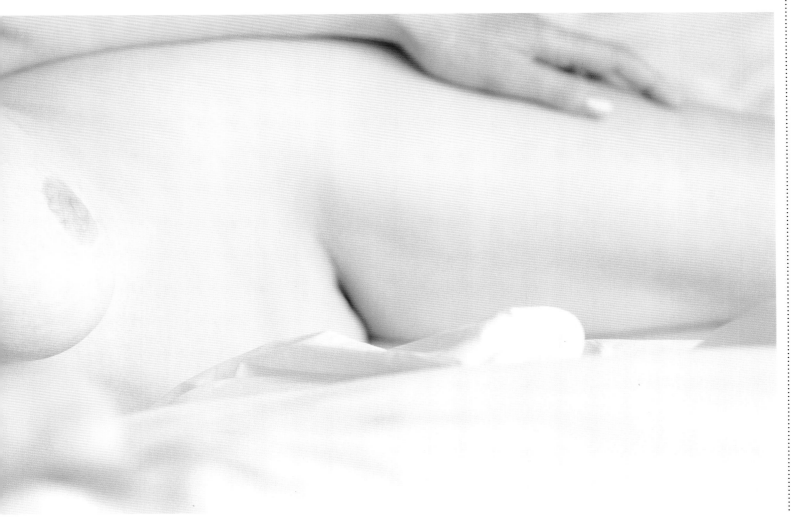

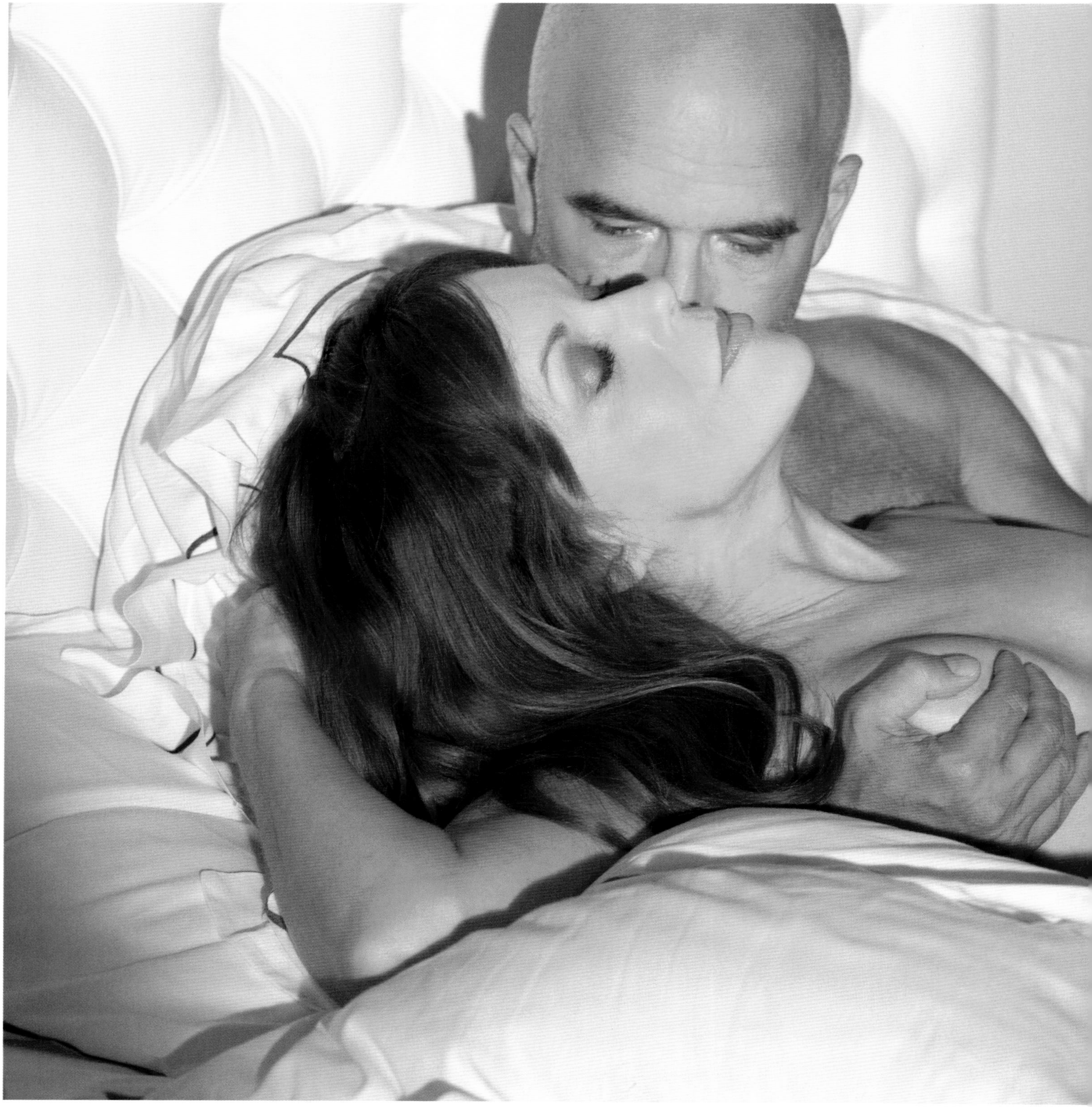

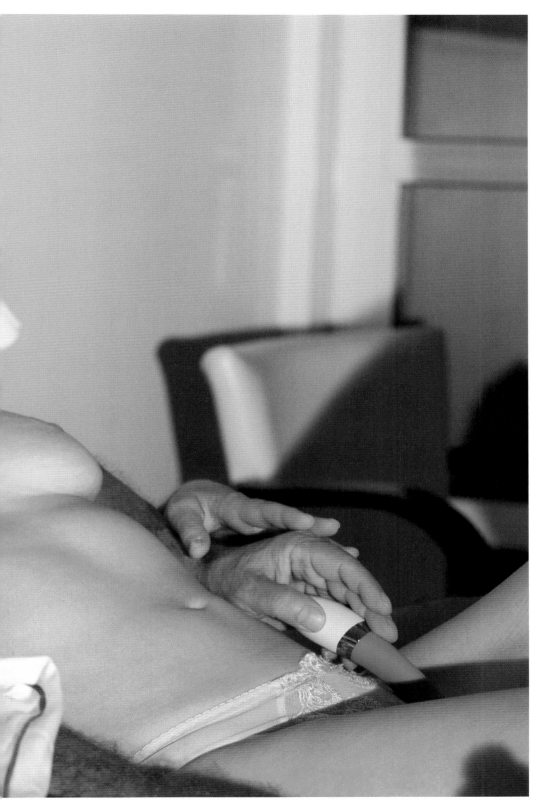

Further, in his book *Younger (Sexier) You: Look and Feel 15 Years Younger by Having the Best Sex of Your Life*, anti-aging expert Eric R. Braverman, M.D., says that sex not only raises your hormone levels, keeping you young, but can also boost your metabolism, brain function, heart health, and immunity.

Still not convinced? Scientists in the School of Social and Community Medicine at the University of Bristol, United Kingdom, conducted a study on the relationship between frequency of orgasm and mortality. They followed more than nine hundred subjects between the ages of forty-five and forty-nine until their deaths. The study found a correlation between the number of orgasms men achieved and lower mortality. In other words, men who have more orgasms live longer, period.

SEX GIVES YOU A WORKOUT

Did you know that 30 minutes of sex burns between 85 and 250 calories? If you have sex three times per week for one year, you could lose 4 pounds (1.8 kg) just by doing what you love. If you're not the type to make regular visits to the gym, then sex could become your new favorite exercise. Without even trying, you'll stretch and tone just about every muscle in your body (including your pelvic muscles, which improves bladder and bowel control). Having sex is a lot more fun than using a treadmill—and you get to control the incline! (Don't cancel your gym membership yet, though. As great as sex is for exercise, regular exercise and healthy eating are still the best ways to control your weight.)

The best ways to get a maximum workout from sex are:

• Go from position to position so that all your muscles get a workout.
• The missionary position works his arms.
• Her gluteal muscles and thighs come into play when she's on top.
• The standing position strengthens both partners' legs.
• In the spooning position, her hips get a good workout.

So mix up your moves and reap the benefits!

SEX IS HEART HEALTHY

As a mature adult, you may be concerned about overexerting yourself or your partner during sex. Midlife adults do in fact face more health risks in general than do their younger peers. However, sex isn't usually considered one of these risks.

People over fifty often express concern that having sex will bring on either a heart attack or stroke. It's even common for couples to avoid having any kind of strenuous sex for fear that something terrible will happen. Although these fears are perfectly understandable, and are rooted in a desire to protect each other, a study by British researchers in the *Journal of Epidemiology and Community Health* found that the frequency of sex was NOT at all associated with strokes in the group of nearly one thousand men that they followed for twenty years. More important, men who had sex at least twice weekly *reduced* their risk of having a fatal heart attack by 50 percent compared with men who had sex less than once a month.

Statistically, only 1 percent of men die of a heart attack during sex. However, it turns out that the vast majority of that 1 percent was having sex with either a mistress or a prostitute at the time. It would appear that the thrill of cheating and potentially being caught, or of having "taboo" sex, might be what puts the ticker into overdrive—not the act itself.

DR. LAURIE'S FIVE-PART SEX STRATEGY

1. Schedule twenty minutes, twice a week, to focus on sexual pleasure.
2. Think of sex as part of your daily workout routine.
3. Focus on the benefits (all the reasons you're committing to this process).
4. Repeat to yourself: "This is really good for me and for us."
5. Just make it happen!

The research is overwhelming: Sex benefits your physical and emotional well-being. Although some of the benefits are obvious, others are simply a bonus. But neglecting your sexual self, however, can have an equally negative effect.

The human body is an efficient machine that requires more attention than a car. You go to the doctor every year for a full physical. You go to the dentist every six months for a cleaning. And you do it because if you neglect your body, bad things happen. It's no different with human sexuality. Mature men who have frequent sex can reduce their risks of prostate problems and difficulties in maintaining an erection. And women who have regular sex are actually helping their bodies produce the hormones responsible for their vaginal health and sexual desire.

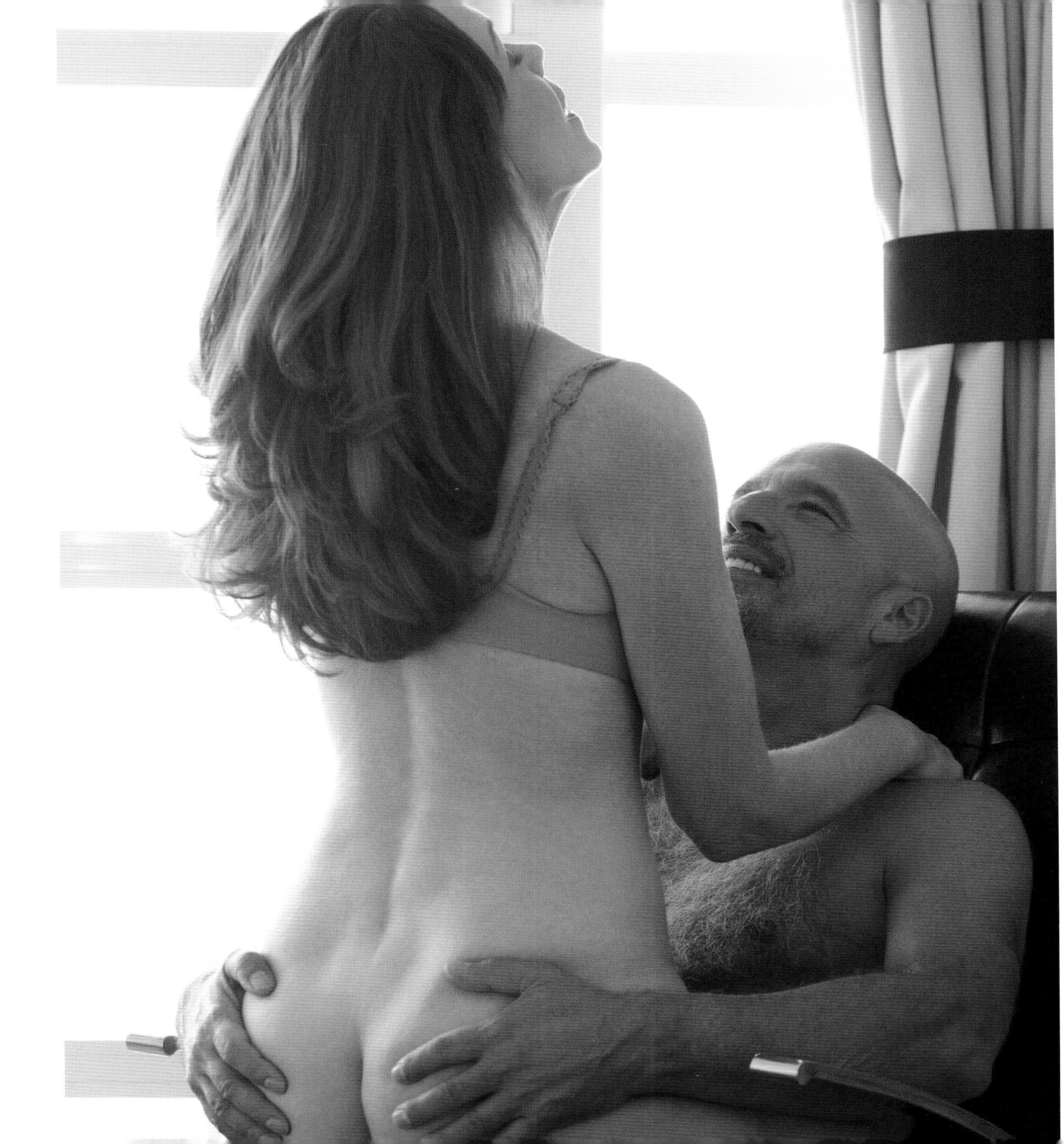

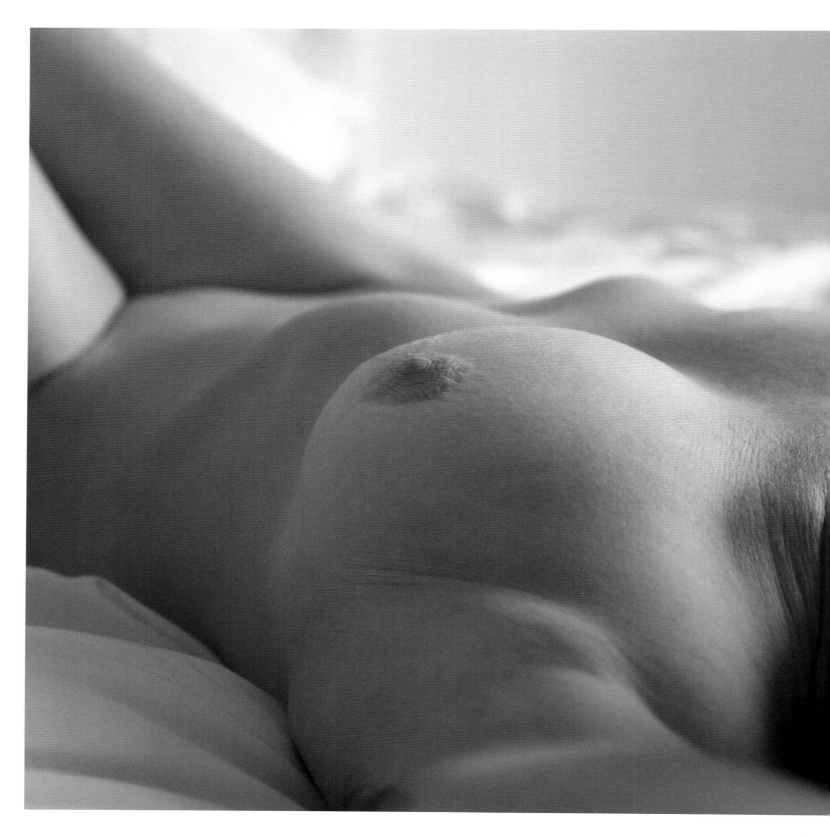

☿ 03 *For the Sultry Woman of a Certain Age*

A forty-nine-year-old woman and her fifty-something husband came to see me because they'd stopped having sex several years before, and when they finally tried again, she found it too painful to continue. It turns out that she didn't have a clue about the effects of menopause. She knew the word, but she didn't know what it meant.

Unfortunately, even members of the medical community may not be up to date on this topic or willing to discuss it. This chapter, then, is for any couple in the same predicament as my clients. Although it focuses on the health and sexuality of a woman as she ages, the information here is beneficial for both partners. It will clear up misconceptions, perhaps tell you some things you didn't know about the topic, and give you easy solutions to common issues.

There's a lot of information about menopause that doctors don't have the chance or time to tell us because they're so rushed. Yet without this information, women can't even formulate the right questions to ask. If you're armed with accurate information about your sexuality at this stage of life, you can make better choices about your body and sexual health—and that allows you to open your mind to all sorts of different possibilities.

However, it's critical that you share new knowledge with your partner, especially about how your body is changing. He's not living in your body, and he has no idea how you feel if you don't tell him. For example, if you avoid having sex because you're experiencing vaginal dryness, he may simply assume you're no longer attracted to him. Too much guesswork hurts relationships.

CELEBRATE MENOPAUSE!

Menopause is the cessation of a woman's menses (her period), which indicates that she can no longer become pregnant. Basically, her ovaries are no longer producing estrogen and progesterone. A woman is considered in menopause when she hasn't had a period for one year.

According to the National Institute on Aging, the average age for menopause is fifty-one. However, symptoms of menopause can be experienced many years earlier and can last months or years after periods stop. A woman is said to be in perimenopause three to five years before menopause, when her estrogen levels begin to decrease.

Menopause is a normal part of life, much like puberty. Having said good-bye to our reproductive years, it's a time when we get to reclaim our sexuality for sexuality's sake. This is good news, because sex is now purely for pleasure.

HELP EASE THE TRANSITION

Not all women seek or even need medical help for symptoms related to menopause, whether they're experiencing hot flashes and night sweats or anxiety and vaginal dryness. The fact is that many women don't experience symptoms severe enough to require treatment. However, if symptoms are affecting your daily life, you should see your family doctor or gynecologist because the more you know about this transition, the better your sex life will be.

Some women fear that their doctors will automatically prescribe hormones. My friend and colleague, Cleve Ziegler, M.D., the director of gynecology of the Jewish General Hospital in Montreal, says, "We don't automatically give menopausal women hormone replacement. We only treat those women who are symptomatic and who have difficulty living with those symptoms." In other words, doctors aren't eager to provide you with hormones, so you should feel safe discussing your options with your physician.

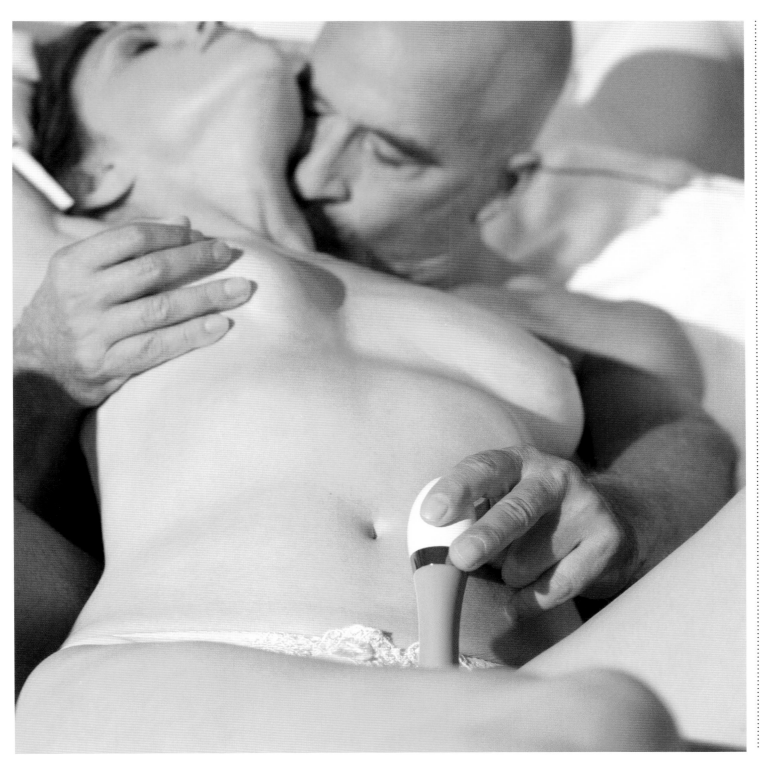

VULVA LOVE

Along with the rest of our bodies, the appearance of our genitals may change with age. For example, the labia (vaginal lips) may darken or droop. For the majority of women, this poses no problem whatsoever and has no effect on sexuality. However, for a small minority of women, labia that hang too loose or droop may make sex uncomfortable if they get pulled during the in-and-out movement of penetration.

Fortunately, there's a fix for that. Some cosmetic surgeons and gynecologists perform a procedure called labiaplasty, in which "extra" labial skin is cut away. In 2006, the American Society of Plastic Surgery reported a little more than one thousand "vaginal rejuvenation" procedures. But unless your genitals are causing you discomfort, labiaplasty is completely unnecessary. I've asked the question about "vaginal beauty" on my radio program for years, and men unanimously say they love all vulvas, period.

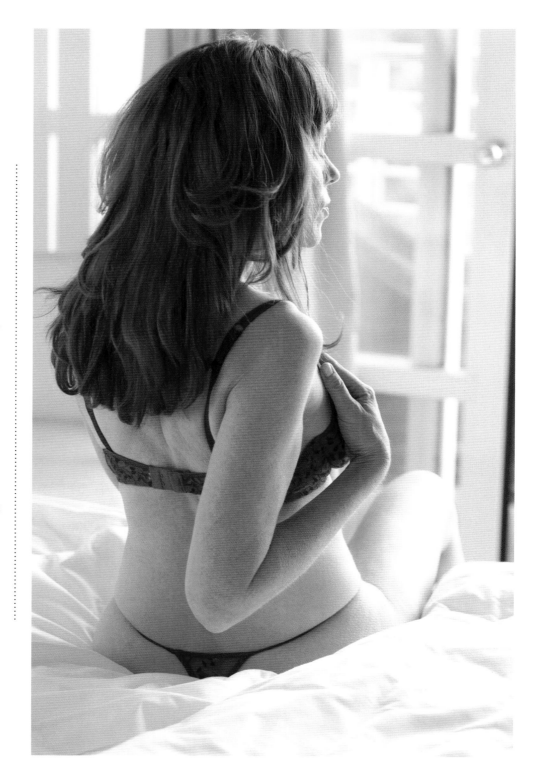

A NOTE ABOUT HRT

Hormone Replacement Therapy (HRT) can relieve menopausal symptoms such as vaginal dryness, vaginal itching, bone-density loss, hot flashes, and night sweats. Although HRT is very good for treating these symptoms (see page 43), it can pose some risks to a woman's overall health. For this reason, doctors tend to prescribe HRT to the few women who are very symptomatic; whereas in the past, it was automatically given to all menopausal women. Only a medical professional can assess your risk factors.

Bottom line: The kind of treatment you should have depends on your symptoms and your medical history. Symptoms are just symptoms. You can STILL have a great and satisfying sex life if you follow some solid advice. You just may have to do things a little differently.

HOW DOES MENOPAUSE AFFECT SEXUALITY?

The symptoms of menopause can begin well before a woman stops menstruating completely. Good news: Most have no effect on your sexuality! However, you *may* notice the following, in various degrees: changes in your sexual response cycle, vaginal atrophy and dryness, or vaginal laxity.

CHANGES IN THE SEXUAL RESPONSE CYCLE

There are several phases to our sexual response, some of which may be affected by aging.

• *Arousal and excitement.* As women (and men) age, they may take longer to reach their excitement phase because less blood is flowing to the genitals. Something similar happens to other areas of our bodies as we age, as well.
Solution: Use a clitoral stimulator to provide more direct contact. Pick one that provides a strong vibration (see chapter 8).

• *Plateau.* Because your body may be producing less vaginal lubrication, your plateau phase—the buildup to orgasm—may take longer.
Solution: Increase foreplay, and during intercourse, apply pressure to your clitoris with a hand or sex toy.

• *Orgasm.* For many women, orgasms become less frequent and less intense after menopause. This could be a result of diminished hormones, medications, or another physical problem related to aging. However, your *ability* to reach orgasm doesn't disappear!
Solution: Let go of orgasm as the goal and enjoy the journey. You can still experience pleasure during sex even if you don't climax, and focusing too much on whether you're going to orgasm can actually reduce the chances that you will.

• *Resolution.* In this phase, your body recuperates.
Solution: Bask in the afterglow!

As you can see, with simple solutions, the changes to your sexual response cycle after "the change" do not make sex any less enjoyable.

VAGINAL ATROPHY

Vaginal inflammation, shrinking, and thinning of the vaginal walls—atrophy—are due to the decline in estrogen that accompanies menopause. According to one Canadian study, 66 percent of postmenopausal women *avoid sexual intimacy because of the fear of painful intercourse caused by vaginal atrophy*. Unfortunately, many women feel uncomfortable discussing this topic with their significant other—or seeking medical help. What a shame, when this is such an easy problem that can be remedied.

Solution: Talk to your partner about your discomfort, as communication is essential. Although having sex is probably the last thing you want to do when your vagina feels irritated and dry, continuous sexual activity is the best way to bring blood to your sexual organs and keep your vaginal walls healthy. Be sure to include foreplay and gentle stimulation, along with a personal lubricant.

VAGINAL DRYNESS

A by-product of vaginal atrophy, vaginal dryness is caused by inadequate lubrication. It may be accompanied by burning and itching, especially during sex. Sadly, it often leads to women flat-out refusing sex, which makes it a big concern for couples.

Lack of vaginal lubrication is NOT necessarily a sign of lack of arousal, especially for women over fifty. Before you assume that you can't possibly be turned on—or that he isn't turning you on—let's find out what your genitals go through as you age and what you can easily do about it.

The walls of the vagina are normally lubricated with a thin layer of fluid. When a woman is sexually aroused, blood flows to her sexual organs, which creates even more fluid. When estrogen levels decrease, as during menopause, the vaginal walls lose their elasticity and become more fragile and vulnerable to small tears. A typical consequence of vaginal dryness is pain—or in more serious cases, bleeding—during sex, along with a burning sensation.

Although vaginal dryness can occur at any age due to different causes—breastfeeding women sometimes experience it, for example—it's most often experienced during or after menopause, and gynecologists report that it's the number-one complaint of women over fifty.

Solution: Fortunately, there are many remedies, prescribed estrogen-based and over-the-counter lubricants being the most accessible and least expensive, that can help restore the necessary lubrication to the vaginal walls, making intercourse pleasurable again. In many instances, a good personal lubricant is all that is needed, but if the problem persists talk to your physician about other options.

What Is Vaginal Laxity?

The term *vaginal laxity* refers to the stretching of the vagina and its opening, the introitus. The condition is generally associated with vaginal delivery or pelvic organ prolapse (dropping of the bladder, uterus, and/or rectum); however, it may also just happen naturally as we age. A woman with this condition might feel "loose," and some may even feel like their insides are going to fall out. This looseness can affect sexual satisfaction, especially if she doesn't feel her partner inside or he isn't getting enough friction during intercourse.

Research into this area is relatively new. In one pilot study, women and their doctors found that the surgery to rectify vaginal laxity, called vaginoplasty—the removal of excess vaginal lining and the tightening of the surrounding soft tissues and muscles— was more effective than simply doing Kegel exercises or undergoing pelvic floor physical therapy, although both are also great options.

Some women may need another type of surgery, called colpoperineorrhaphy, to repair the area; it's akin to an episiotomy repair. A third study found that nonsurgical radiofrequency thermal therapy, which is basically microwaves applied to the tissues to tighten the skin, was an effective treatment: Patients reported a significant improvement in vaginal tightness and sexual function, as well as decreased sexual distress. Research in this area is ongoing, so try to stay informed of new developments!

What If I'm Too Tight?

With age—especially if you've had a hysterectomy, reconstructive surgery for prolapse, or radiation for cancer treatment— the length of the vagina shortens, and the opening may narrow. This may cause pain during intercourse. If you're experiencing this, don't despair! Discuss your options with your gynecologist; several treatment methods are available, such as physical therapy, the use of vaginal dilators, or even surgery.

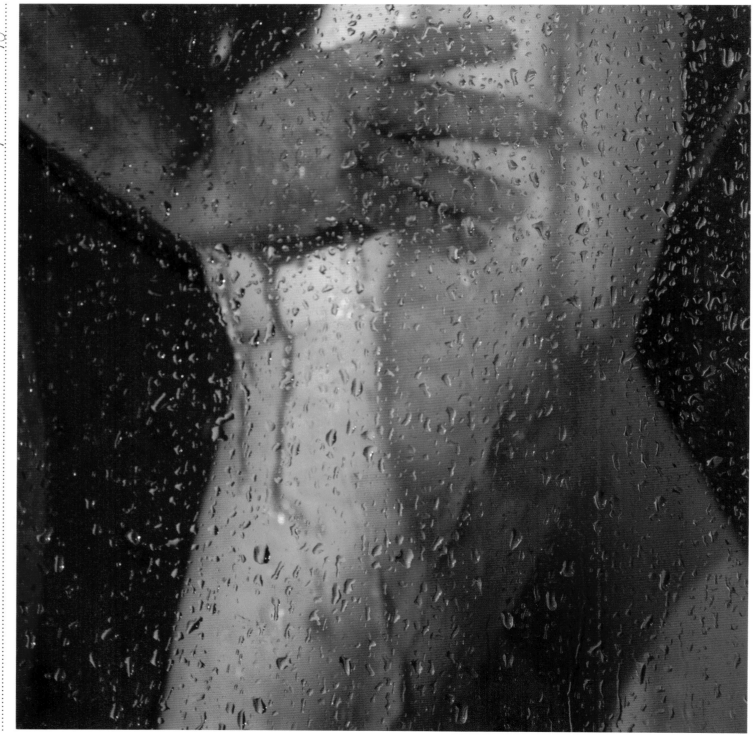

Hormone Replacement Therapy
Hormone replacement therapy, or HRT, is one viable option for menopausal women experiencing vaginal dryness. Talk to your doctor about whether this is right for you.

Topical forms of HRT have become the first line of defense. They include:
• Creams that are applied in the vagina with an applicator, such as Premarin.
• Vaginal estrogen rings that are inserted into the upper part of the vagina, such as Estring.
• Vaginal estrogen tablets that are also inserted into the vagina, such as Vagifem.

But if topical forms aren't the right solution for you, there are systemic forms that also provide the body with estrogen replacement. The difference is that topical forms used in the vagina do not, for the most part, enter your bloodstream. The systemic forms such as skin patches (such as Alora) or oral medications (such as Estrace) do. That being said, in general, women report that topical therapy is more effective for treating vaginal dryness than hormones taken orally or by skin patch.

Local Estrogen Therapy (LET)
This hormonal option is estrogen that is applied directly in the vagina via a tablet, ring, or cream, to help restore vaginal tissue. It's a wonderfully effective medication for treating vaginal dryness and discomfort during intercourse, and it has fewer risks than HRT. As a bonus, it also helps with urinary problems. The Society of Obstetricians and Gynecologists of Canada highly recommends LET as the most appropriate treatment for vaginal atrophy. Usually a week of daily use, followed by an application every few days, will ease symptoms, and you'll start experiencing less-painful intercourse within a few weeks of treatment. As always, discuss this option with your medical practitioner.

Over-the-Counter Vaginal Lubricants
If you aren't comfortable with the idea of HRT or if you simply want to deal with vaginal dryness in a non-hormonal way, vaginal lubricants are a great solution. Sold as "personal lubricants," usually in the "feminine needs" section of the grocery store or drugstore, lubricants can augment or replace the fluid normally created by blood flow during sexual activity and can significantly reduce pain during intercourse. Water-based products are less likely to cause allergic reactions, whereas silicone-based products last longer but also feel much "greasier" and take longer to dry out. Take the time to find the right lubricant for you. Don't be afraid to try out different kinds.

A note of caution: Use only water-based lubricants if you're using condoms, as oil-based lubricants deteriorate latex.

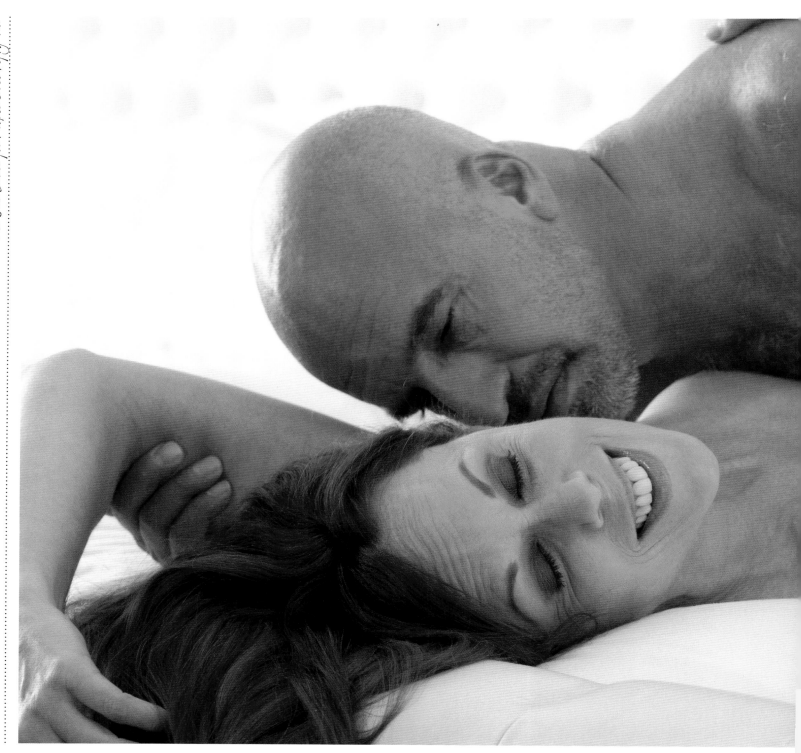

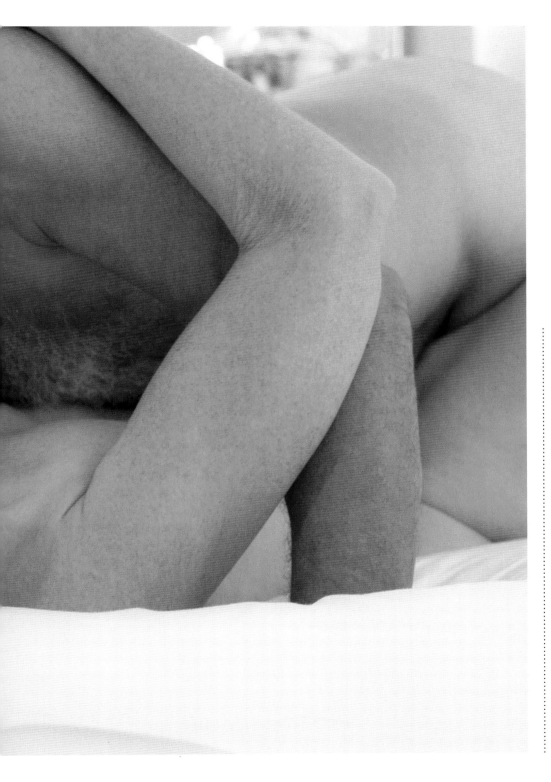

IT'S NOT JUST MENOPAUSE

Factors other than menopause can exacerbate or trigger vaginal dryness. Some of these culprits include the following:

Douching disrupts the normal chemical balance in the vagina, which can lead to dryness and irritation.

Medications that contain decongestants decrease the moisture in your body, which could therefore lead to vaginal dryness.

Anti-estrogen medications, such as those used to treat breast cancer, can cause vaginal dryness because they reduce the estrogen needed to keep the vaginal walls healthy.

Lack of foreplay before intercourse may not give the vagina time to lubricate. The body needs stimulation to get the juices flowing!

EXERCISES TO GET YOUR GROOVE BACK

Pelvic floor muscles, including the pubococcygeus (PC) muscle, are important for keeping the genital area strong and healthy. These muscles can weaken as we age, so it's important to strengthen them to maximize sexual pleasure. In fact, research since the 1950s has repeatedly shown that doing regular Kegel exercises (described in the next section) helps women achieve better, stronger orgasms. By creating a tighter vaginal canal, these exercises help a woman better feel her man's girth. This tightness will invariably increase his pleasure as well! As a bonus, performing pelvic floor exercises can help with another common complaint of aging: the leaky bladder.

Kegel Exercises

The most famous pelvic floor exercises are Kegel exercises, in which you contract and then relax the pelvic floor muscles. To locate those muscles, try stopping the flow of urine midstream. Squeeze, and then let go. (Do this only to find the muscles. Afterward, practice the exercise outside the bathroom walls.) Try to avoid flexing the gluteal, thigh, or abdominal muscles.

You can begin doing Kegels by contracting your pelvic floor muscles for 5 seconds and then releasing them for 5 seconds. Do this a few times in a row. Ideally, you should repeat this exercise three times a day and, once you're used to it, aim to keep your muscles contracted for 10 seconds at a time. Kegel exercises are discreet. You can do them anytime, anywhere, and no one will notice! Do the following Kegel exercise program three times a day anywhere, anytime, clothed or not:

• Do three sets of 15 repetitions each time.
• First set: Squeeze for 3 seconds and then release. Repeat 15 times.
• Second set: Contract and release quickly. Repeat 15 times.
• Third set: Alternate between a quick contraction and a long (3-second) squeeze.
• Couple Kegels: Practice during sexual intercourse, with both partners alternately contracting and releasing.

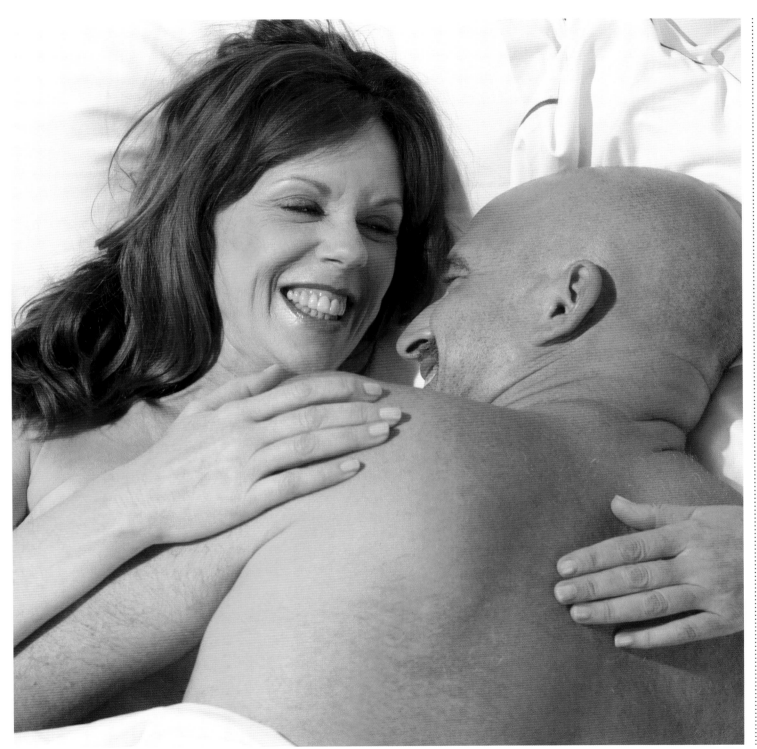

EXERCISE YOUR BODY AND YOUR SEXUALITY WILL FOLLOW

....

While we're on the topic of exercises, it turns out that the more you exercise your entire body, the more you'll enjoy sex! That's the conclusion of a 2010 study published in *The European Journal of Contraception & Reproductive Health Care*. Researchers found that premenopausal women who reported higher levels of physical activity also reported better sex. Premenopausal women who were less active reported decreased sexual desire, decreased arousal and lubrication, fewer orgasms, and less satisfaction. It's never too late to get the blood flowing. Go for a nice brisk evening walk with your partner and get your blood pumping. You may find that you want to keep it pumping all the way into your bedroom.

....

Pelvic Floor Physical Therapy

Many of my patients who complain of pain during intercourse have found that pelvic floor physical therapy helps them control their pain and has not only made intercourse possible, but also more enjoyable. It's a relatively new specialty that involves working manually with the whole pelvic region. The physical therapist uses her hands, a probe, or a dilator in a woman's vagina to help her gain control of her vaginal muscles. This is a great option if you have weak pelvic floor muscles, as the physical therapist stimulates the muscles with various techniques to strengthen them. She may also suggest electrical muscle stimulation or teach you manual techniques that you can do at home.

The exercises you'll learn with a specialized physical therapist are different than regular Kegels. Here, a health care professional will work directly with your genitals to get the muscles working properly. She'll show you—through biofeedback techniques, for example—different ways to do the exercises. Yes, they use a "hands-on" approach, which you may or may not be comfortable with; however, for some women, this approach is very effective. (Think of it as similar to a visit to the gynecologist.)

Because this is such a new area of study, ask your gynecologist for a recommendation, ask a physical therapist whether she treats the pelvic floor, or turn to the Web to find a women's health physical therapist.

Ben-Wa Balls

Ben-Wa balls are weighted balls, usually made of metal, that you insert into your vagina and try to keep from falling out by contracting your PC muscle (that is, do a Kegel) almost continuously. This is another great way to exercise your vagina.

Ben-Wa balls come in different sizes, and sometimes in different forms—a Google search will turn up dozens of examples. Often they have a string attached, and many women experience pleasure when they finally pull them out. Since the erotic novel *Fifty Shades of Grey* came out, the sale of Ben-Wa balls has skyrocketed. (The main character inserts them into her vagina and then proceeds to keep them in during most of her date.) Give them a try!

MENOPAUSE DOES NOT DAMPEN LIBIDO

Let's get one final worry out of the way: Menopause does not have to decrease your sex drive. It might even increase your libido now that you're no longer worried about getting pregnant!

In fact, psychological and emotional factors are more likely to cool a woman's interest in sex than treatable physical conditions are. These factors include resentment toward her partner and the feeling that the relationship has grown monotonous, boring, or routine. Conversely, many studies have found that women who have a positive outlook on their relationships and partners report higher levels of sexual satisfaction.

So, if you want to rekindle your sexual feelings, going through menopause won't stop you. It's about the actions you take—such as the ones covered in this book—and your overall attitude.

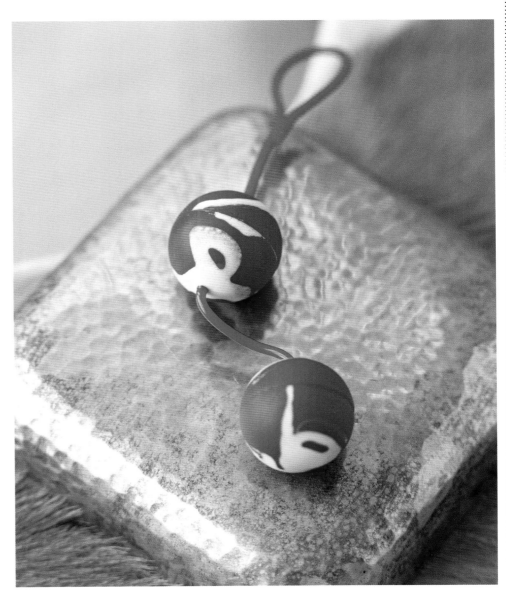

Ben-Wa Balls

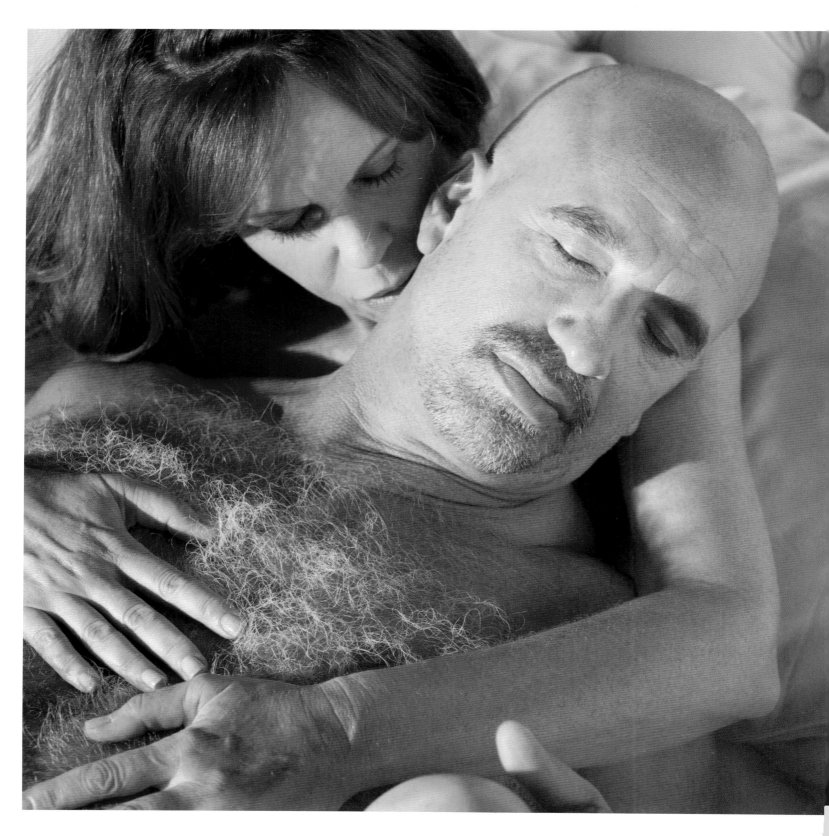

♂4 *For the Distinguished Man*

All men experience changes in their sexuality as they age. It just happens at different times for different men. For some, the changes show up at thirty-five, but others don't notice anything until they're in their sixties. They might observe that their erections hang at a lower angle or are less rigid. They might take longer to orgasm, and when it happens, they ejaculate less and not as forcefully as before. Their refractory period—the recovery period before they can have another orgasm—might be longer, too.

Despite these changes, the majority of mature men still report satisfying sex lives. Armed with accurate information about treatment options (if and when necessary), specific strategies, and a positive attitude, you and your partner will find that sex after fifty can be better than it's ever been!

"MAN-OPAUSE"

Andropause, aka "man-opause" or testosterone deficiency syndrome, is as close to the equivalent of menopause that men have. It refers to the period—which can occur any time between the ages of forty and fifty-five—when men begin to exhibit signs that their testosterone and other hormone levels are dropping. Unlike women, who know when they are menopausal because their periods stop, men seem to transition slowly into this phase, which can span several decades.

Although all women go through menopause, not all men will experience andropausal symptoms. According to Michael Werner, M.D., a well-known urologist and specialist in sexual dysfunction who's written extensively on this subject, about 2 to 5 percent of forty- to forty-nine-year-old men experience andropause, whereas by age sixty, the likelihood is somewhere between 20 and 40 percent.

Until recently, andropause went undiagnosed and untreated, and it was often confused with other conditions. The good news is that today we have better methods to detect hormone levels, and thus the medical community is talking more openly about it.

Remember, not all men will experience symptoms to a degree that they find bothersome! So far, we don't have any way to predict who will suffer some of the more severe symptoms—or when.

ANDROPAUSE SYMPTOMS AND THEIR IMPACT ON SEX

Andropausal symptoms may occur quite gradually. They include:

• *Changes in attitudes and moods.* This can have you feeling depressed and irritable, which will make you less likely to want to have sex, and will likely have your partner avoiding you.

• *Fatigue and loss of energy.* Being chronically tired stamps out our flame—and leaves us with little energy for the fun stuff.

• *Loss of physical agility and strength.* You may find it difficult to also keep up your sexual stamina.

• *Loss of sex drive.* You will feel like you have lost your "mojo."

• *A decrease in the strength of erections.* You may get erections, but they will not be as rigid as before.

Some men find they start falling asleep right after dinner. Others find that they're not able to play the sports they had once mastered, or that their work performance is slipping. They may simply experience decreased enjoyment in life.

The word *andropause* –sometimes called testosterone deficiency syndrome or man-opause–comes from the Latin *andro*, meaning "male." It's a fairly new term, and the condition itself isn't well understood.

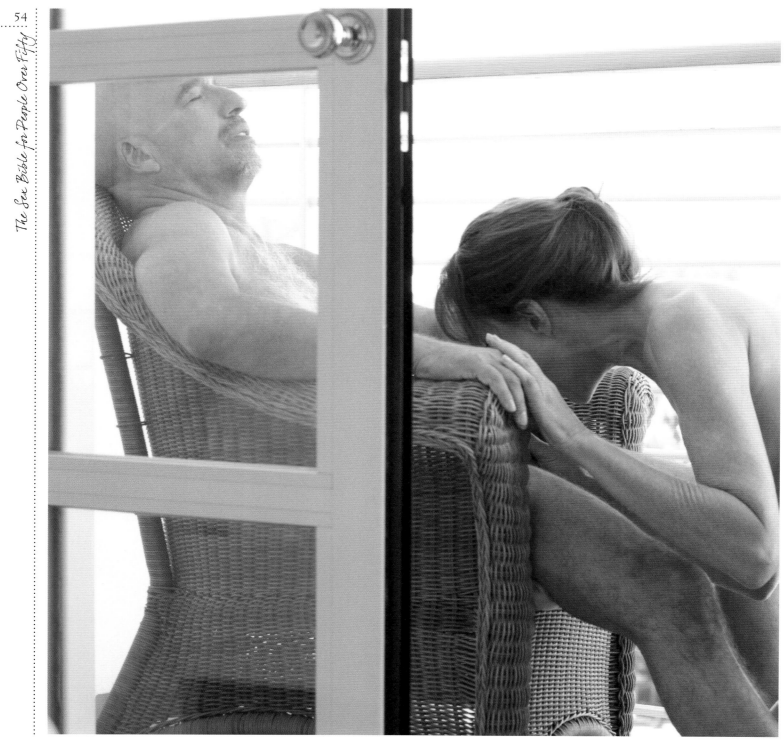

HOW TO SPOT IT IF YOU'VE GOT IT

The two markers of andropause that physicians tend to use most are decreased sex drive and erectile difficulties. If you're having these or any of the other symptoms mentioned here, there's a likelihood you have low testosterone and should be checked by a physician. A simple blood test can help determine testosterone levels. Please note: Not all men will experience all symptoms with the same severity! The symptoms listed are worst-case scenarios. But if they're affecting your sexuality, talk to your doctor about your options to get back in the groove. By addressing your sex life, you'll reduce other health risks of andropause. For example, decreased hormone levels have been associated with osteoporosis and cardiovascular disease in both men and women. As discussed in chapter 2, an active sex life helps with overall health.

HORMONES TO THE RESCUE

Testosterone replacement therapy is the treatment of choice for men whose levels are low as shown by a blood test measuring "free" or "bioavailable" testosterone. In simple terms, most of the testosterone we have in our blood is bound to a protein called sex hormone binding globulin (SHBG). The remaining 40 percent of the testosterone that is not bound, however, is referred to as "bioavailable," and is mostly responsible for our sexual functioning.

The bioavailable test is the most accurate, but not all labs perform it, so be sure to specify to your doctor that you want this particular blood test. Men who respond well to hormone treatment report feeling revitalized, energized, and ready for sex. Some of the other benefits include increased muscle mass, improved memory and concentration, increased libido, better sleep, and increased motivation.

THE TRUTH ABOUT MEN OVER FORTY AND ERECTILE DYSFUNCTION

In a 2003 Canadian sexual satisfaction survey of more than 4,500 men aged forty and over:

34 percent were found to have erectile dysfunction (ED)

83 percent of men with ED were at least still somewhat satisfied with their sex life

73 percent of men with ED had sex 4.4 times per month on average (vs. 7.3 for men without ED)

54 percent dealt easily with the ED with their partner

97 percent reported their partner was completely understanding

There are several testosterone replacement treatment options including:
• Intramuscular injections
• Testosterone patch
• Testosterone gel
• Oral tablets
• Long-acting subcutaneous implant

Each treatment has different advantages and disadvantages. Talk to your doctor to see which approach may be right for you. Before you can start testosterone replacement therapy and get your soldier saluting again, you first have to see your doctor so he or she can order the blood test! Don't be shy about discussing andropause with your physician. He or she may not ask you questions about your sex life unless you bring it up. You need to be your own advocate. And isn't your sex life worth it?

ED: WHAT YOU NEED TO KNOW

The symptom that most often leads men to seek treatment is ED, defined as the inability to achieve or sustain an erection that's hard enough or lasts long enough to complete sexual intercourse or another sexual activity. The truth is that *most* men at *some* point in their lives experience an occasional failure to get an erection due to stress, fatigue, anxiety, or alcohol. When this happens, it's nothing to worry about.

Aging will also affect the rigidity of your erections. It takes longer to achieve an erection, and men need more direct stimulation to stay hard. If this happens to you, you probably don't need treatment. *Sex strategy:* Spend more time on foreplay, especially oral sex or manual stimulation.

For about 25 percent of men, however, erectile problems are severe enough that they require medical intervention.

MEDICAL ISSUES AND ED

Terry Mason, M.D., chief medical officer at Cook County Health and Hospitals System in Chicago and a prominent expert in the field of ED, believes that the problem is a leading indicator of heart disease. If you experience ED regularly (in other words, more than on one occasion), see your doctor and get a full medical checkup as soon as possible. Early diagnosis and treatment can save your life.

If you suffer from any of these conditions, you're more likely to experience ED:
• Alcoholism
• Clogged blood vessels
• Diabetes
• Heart disease
• High blood pressure
• High cholesterol
• Mental health issues such as depression, anxiety, stress, and relationship problems
• Multiple sclerosis
• Parkinson's disease
• Prostate cancer or enlarged prostate

TREATMENT OPTIONS FOR ED

If you're experiencing ED, don't despair! There are a number of options to treat this condition. Discuss them with your doctor, who will tailor a course of treatment to your specific needs.

Oral Medications

Oral medications for ED are the treatment of choice for many men. I'm sure you've heard the trade names: Viagra, Cialis, Levitra, and Staxyn. These drugs enhance the effects of nitric oxide, which is found in your body and relaxes the muscles in your penis. When the muscles are relaxed, more blood flows to the penis and leads to an erection—if and only if you're sexually stimulated. No stimulation, no erection.

These medications don't come without caveats, however. They might not work the first time you use them, and you may need to try each of them until you find the one that suits you best. Common side effects that you need to be aware of include headache, redness or flushing of the face and neck, indigestion, stuffy nose, and "blue vision" (everything seems to have a blue tint to it). None of these side effects is permanent. Check with your doctor to make sure you're a good candidate for these medications and that they won't interfere with any other prescriptions you're taking.

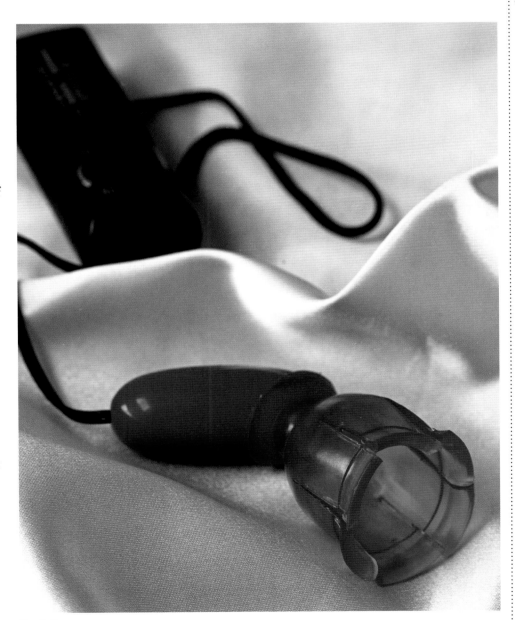

Penile Pump

Understand that occasional ED is common in all men and is not an indicator that it no longer works! Take the time to focus on other sexual activities that do not involve the penis. Turn your attention to pleasuring your partner with your hands and mouth, with no pressure to have intercourse. Try this approach for the next five times you are intimate together.

If you get a prescription from your doctor for any ED medications, don't buy them online. (Some people even try to get these medications without a prescription online.) Research has shown that what's often sold online as Viagra (or the others), really isn't, even if it looks like it. It's a knock-off that may not even contain traces of the necessary ingredient, sildenafil. According to a study presented at the American Urological Association 2012 Annual Scientific Meeting and reported by Irwin Goldstein, M.D., 77 percent of pills sold online were counterfeit.

Also, beware of "natural" remedies. Many nutritional supplements are sold with the promise of improving erections. Sometimes they work, sometimes they don't. The problem is that the Food and Drug Administration doesn't regulate these supplements, and that's because much of what's sold hasn't been through rigorous scientific studies.

Another issue is that if you "self-prescribe" a supplement, you risk not getting to the root of what's causing the ED. If, for example, the cause of your ED is arterial blockages, then you may miss a potentially life-threatening problem. Natural remedies can also interfere with other medications you're taking, so use caution with anything you take, "natural" or not, and check first with your doctor or pharmacist.

Penile Injection

It's not as scary as it sounds. In his book, *A Mind of Its Own: A Cultural History of the Penis*, author David Friedman describes how injections to the penis came to be introduced as a treatment option. An English physiologist by the name of Giles Brindley was working on drugs that, when injected into the penis, would produce erections lasting for several hours, even in men who were paralyzed. At a 1983 urology convention, he made a spectacle of himself by showing his own freshly injected penis to the audience to prove his point!

Since that time, penile injections have been a safe treatment option for men—as safe as other ED treatments, although all options have potential side effects—and a good option for men who do not respond to oral medications. Since the introduction of oral medications, however, this option is not widely used.

With this method, men are taught how to inject alprostadil (sometimes sold under the brand name Caverject) into the base or side of the penis, using a very thin needle. Each injection generally produces an erection within minutes and that lasts about an hour. Unlike a medication such as Viagra, which requires the man to be in the mood and sexually aroused, penile injection works directly on the penile muscles and arteries—no direct stimulation is necessary.

In a study reported in the urology journal *BJU International*, patients comparing this method to the use of sildenafil (Viagra, etc.) found that the hardness of their erection was better with the injection, and the majority of these men wanted to continue using the injection method. Possible side effects include scarring, priapism (prolonged painful erection), bleeding, and bruising.

Intraurethral Suppository

Another treatment for ED involves using a special applicator to insert a suppository containing alprostadil (known under the trade name Muse) into the urethra. An erection usually occurs within 10 minutes that will last between 30 and 60 minutes. Reported side effects include pain, dizziness, and priapism, but only in a negligible number of users. According to the Center for Male Reproductive Medicine and Microsurgery, this method has a 30 to 40 percent success rate (measured by the ability to achieve an erection that is rigid enough for penetration).

Vacuum Erection Device
(or Penis Pump)

Generally sold in sex boutiques and by medical supply companies, this device is a hollow tube with a hand- or battery-powered pump. A man places his penis inside the tube, then uses the pump to create a vacuum by sucking out the air inside the tube, pulling blood into the penis. Once he gets an erection, he removes the device and immediately slips a tension ring (also known as a "cock ring") around the base of his penis to hold in the blood and keep the erection. (He should remove the ring no more than 30 minutes later, which affords plenty of time for intercourse.) Using one of these rings doesn't affect the ability to orgasm, but may impede ejaculation. Other possible side effects include bruising, pain, and penile numbness (all of which are temporary). According to the Weill Cornell Medical College's Department of Urology, satisfaction rates for this device are over the 80 percent mark.

If you're having difficulty maintaining an erection, it doesn't mean that you can't feel— or give—sexual pleasure. If your partner wants the feeling of penetration, try using a dildo on her while you continue to caress her with your free hand.

Penile Implants

This ED treatment is the most invasive and least common option, but the one with the most reported satisfaction from couples. In a study published in the *Journal of Urology*, patient and partner satisfaction was very high (91 percent for men and 83 percent for women). Having said that, consider it only if all other methods have failed.

This surgical method is the treatment of choice, albeit an uncommon one, for men who do not respond to any other treatment option and who have a clear medical cause for their ED. According to Coloplast, the company that distributes penile prosthetic devices, 20,000 such surgeries are performed worldwide each year. Yet, a 2011 study published in the *Journal of Sexual Medicine* reports that penile implants following surgery for prostate cancer was chosen by only 0.8 percent of patients.

The process involves surgically placing rods into each side of the penis. The rods can be either inflatable—where the man squeezes a pump placed in his scrotum whenever he wants an erection—or semi-rigid, where the penis stays firm at all times (but can be bent down when not "in use"). Penile implants do not affect ability to ejaculate. Potential risks include infection and implant malfunction.

Sex Therapy or Psychotherapy

If your penile problems are caused by stress, anxiety, or depression, consider consulting a therapist, either alone or with your partner. Similarly, some medications used to treat these conditions can interfere with penile performance. Relief can come from something as simple as a switch in medications, so talk to your doctor or therapist about all your options.

OTHER PHYSICAL CONCERNS—AND WHAT TO DO ABOUT THEM

Andropause and ED aren't the only sexual issues that men face as they pass fifty. Similar to the physical changes women undergo as they travel through menopause, men's sexual anatomy goes through its own set of alterations.

If your scrotum sags, your partner is most likely to feel your testicles slamming against her while you thrust during the rear-entry and missionary positions. Most women don't mind, but if you feel self-conscious about it, try the female-on-top position, or side-to-side while lying down.

Sagging Scrotum

No one gets older and escapes sagging skin somewhere—and that includes the genitals. If your testicles are hanging low and you're self-conscious about it, a simple procedure called a scrotal lift can remedy the situation. It's an outpatient surgical procedure that's generally done in a hospital (or a clinic that has an operating room) under local anesthesia. It takes from 30 minutes to an hour to perform. Similar to labiaplasty in women, this is elective cosmetic surgery, as there is no medical reason to "fix" this.

Curvature of the Penis

While some curvature of the penis is normal, it may become more pronounced with age. Men whose penises don't stand up completely straight have no issues with intercourse. Sometimes they simply have to maneuver their bodies a little to have easier access to the vagina.

However, a study published in the *International Journal of Impotence Research* reported that approximately 3 to 4 percent of men will suffer from Peyronie's disease—a curvature of the penis that is very pronounced and can cause pain with erections. The risk of acquiring this disease increases with age.

This condition results from a buildup of scar tissue that may have been caused by trauma or injury to the penis, often through rigorous sexual activity (though you may never have been aware that you injured yourself). This scar tissue may cause pain and abnormal curvature of the penis when it's erect. The angle of the penis may make intercourse painful or difficult, but not all men with this condition have problems with sex.

If you notice that your erections cause a big curvature, and it causes you pain, consult a urologist. There's no reason for you to live with penile pain if it can be helped. Depending on the severity, doctors treat this condition with medication, devices to stretch the penis (penis extenders), or surgery.

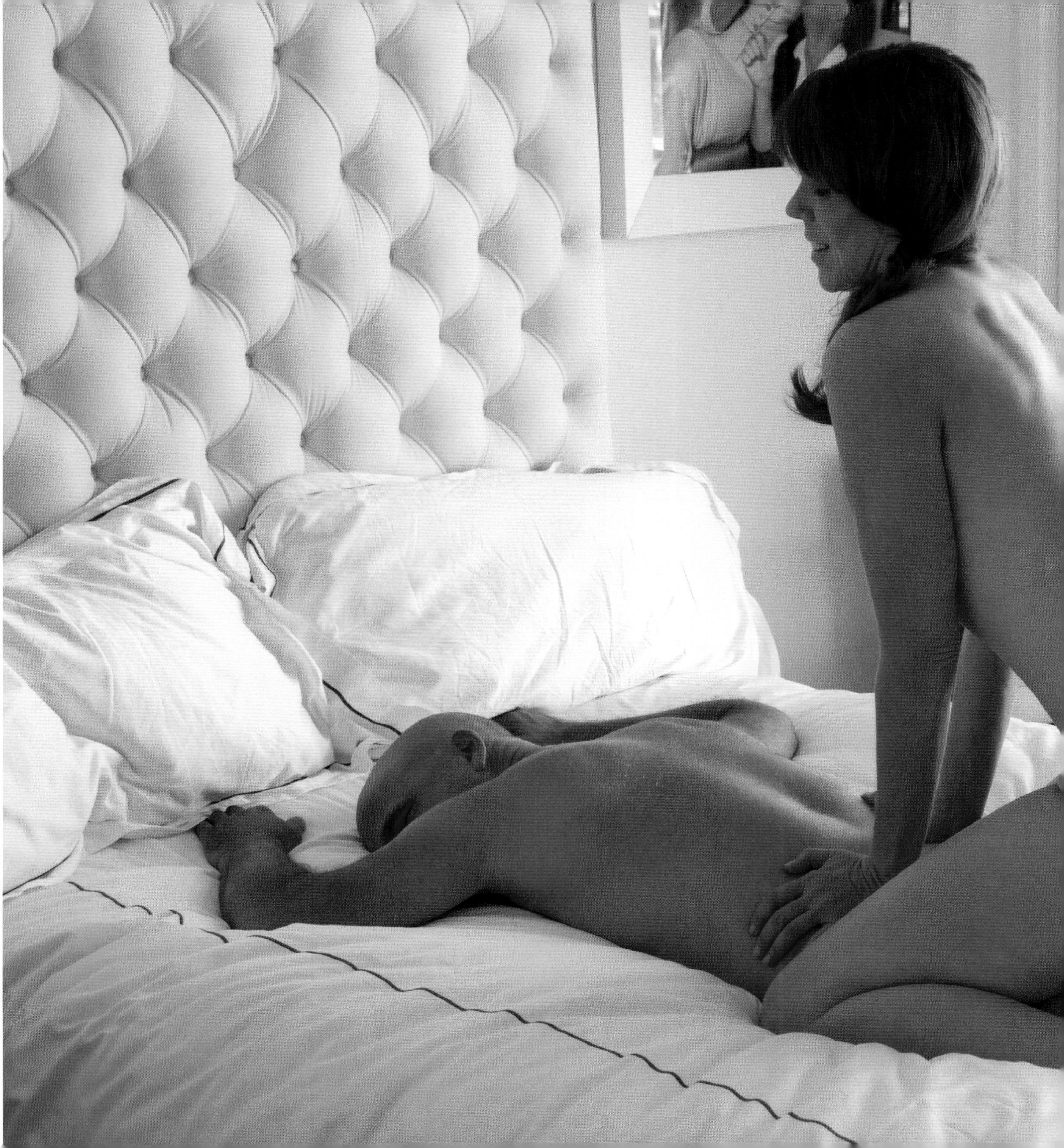

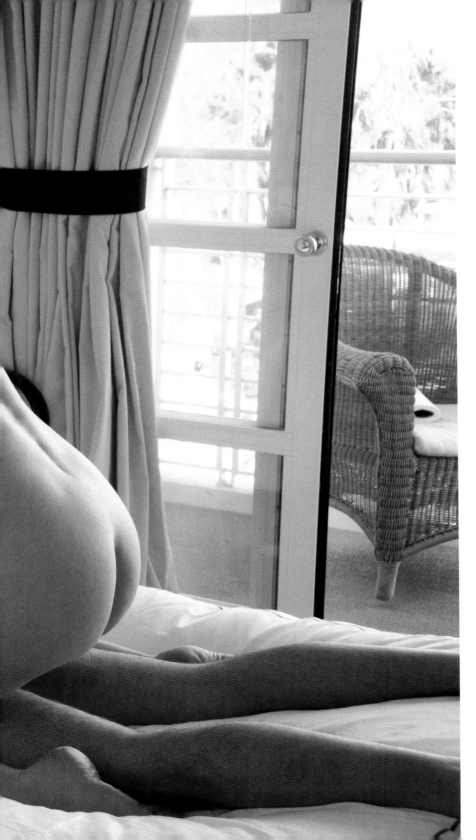

If your penis has developed a slight curve, you may want to have your partner be on top during intercourse so that she can hold your penis and guide it into her vagina. You may have to move your hips a little differently during thrusting. Experiment a little to see what feels comfortable for both of you.

Kegels Are Good for Men, Too!

Studies have shown that doing regular Kegel exercises can help improve the strength of your erection. It can also be effective for men who struggle with premature ejaculation. Strong PC muscles have been associated with stronger, more intense ejaculations and improved bladder control, and have been used in the treatment of prostate difficulties. Use the following Kegel exercise program every day:

• Stand up while urinating and, about halfway through, stop the flow. If you stop it successfully, you have the right muscle.

• Start and stop the flow of urine once or twice during urination to get used to which muscle should be tightened.

• Then, when you're not urinating, practice tightening and relaxing this muscle five to ten times a day, a few minutes at a time, any time of day—ideally, when sitting down.

• Try not to squeeze your buttocks or leg muscles. Instead, focus on the muscles in your pelvic area.

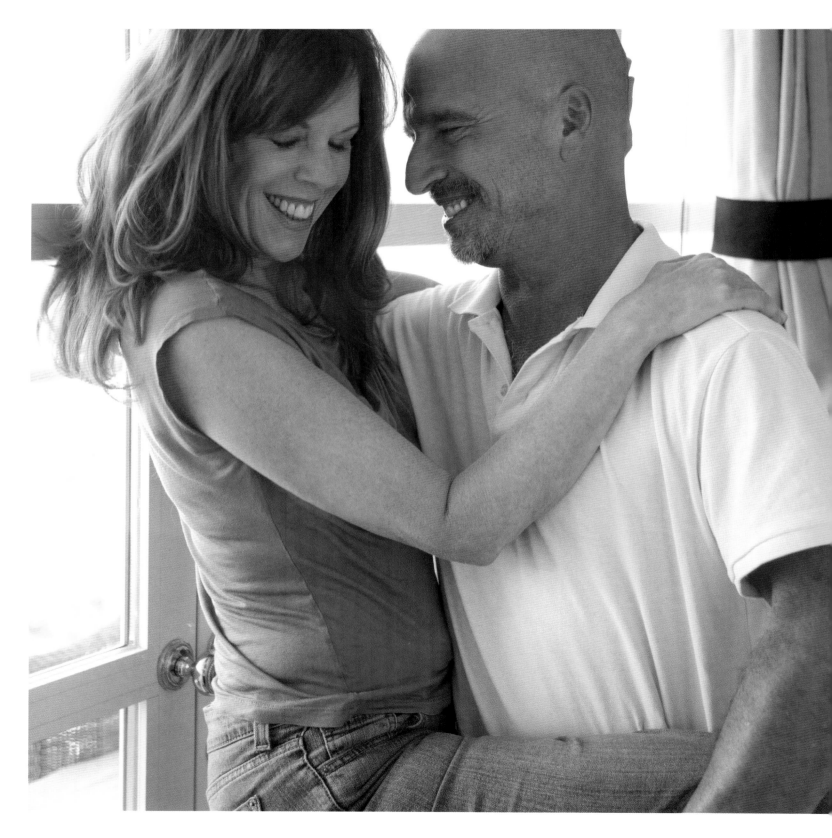

☿5 *Sexual Desire Uncovered*

Sexual desire—also known as libido—is often misunderstood. For one thing, it doesn't stay constant over your life span. If it has remained unchanged, consider yourself a member of the minority! But if you had a strong libido once and now you think that it's just vanished, you're probably feeling troubled and confused. Part of the confusion is that you don't quite understand what happened to your desire. After all, you still love your partner, you still find him or her attractive even after fifteen, twenty, thirty or more years together, and your relationship is solid. So what exactly is the problem? That's what this chapter will uncover for you.

WHAT IS SEXUAL DESIRE?

Sexual desire is the wanting of sexual activity. It's also the thinking about sex. And it's a feeling that can be triggered by internal cues, such as fantasies, or external cues, such as images. Stephen Levine, M.D., author of a number of books and scientific papers on sexuality, describes, in the *Archives of Sexual Behavior*, sexual desire as having three major components:
• *Drive* is what we describe as an urge—something that happens biologically.
• *Motivation* is the psychological component of desire and is influenced by factors such as mood, interpersonal contact, and relationship factors.
• *Wish* is the cultural component of desire, where factors such as values, social rules, and mores influence our state of desire.

To illustrate these components—and the problem that many couples over fifty face—here's a typical example from my practice. Julie, a fifty-two-year-old mother of three who's been married for twenty-three years, came to see me recently. Our conversation went something like this:

Julie: "I have zero desire for sex. I love my husband, but I just don't want sex. He wants it often and thinks there's something seriously wrong with me. So what is wrong with me?"

Me: "When you see a hot guy on screen or in magazines, does it do something to you? Do you ever think about sex during the day? Do you ever feel aroused when reading a sexual passage in a book?"

Julie: "Yes, yes, and yes."

Me: "So you don't get 'horny,' but you're triggered by sexual content?"

Julie: "That's it!"

Me: "When you do have sex, do you feel pleasure?"

Julie: "When we do it, I definitely enjoy it."

Sound familiar?

Julie hasn't lost her interest in sex, just her spontaneous desire for it. So she may not have the *drive*, or the urge, but that doesn't mean she has lost her *motivation* or *wish* for sex. Nor has she lost her ability to be aroused. Desire can definitely be triggered, as long as the motivation and wish for it are there.

One of my favorite speakers and authors on relationships is Pat Love, Ed.D., a sex and love educator. She talks about each of us having a "set point" of desire. We generally fall into one of three categories: low, medium, or high. This set point can be affected by various factors, such as age and gender.

AGING AND DESIRE

Society seems to believe that sexual desire inevitably declines with age, which leads people to assume that sex will stop happening altogether as we get older. Nothing could be further from the truth! According to *The Starr-Weiner Report on Sex and Sexuality in the Mature Years*, age typically doesn't significantly diminish either the need or the desire for sex. Regular sexual activity is the norm when people have a partner, and adults over the age of sixty believe that sex contributes to physical and emotional health.

FEMALE DESIRE AFTER FIFTY

However, one persistent myth is that female sexual desire declines dramatically with age. In fact, the opposite is often true—following menopause, many women experience *more* desire. "Desire, once quelled by birth control pills, could even resurge," says Amanda Richards, M.D., associate professor of obstetrics and gynecology at the University of Miami Miller School of Medicine.

And Margaret E. Wierman, M.D., a professor of medicine, physiology, and biophysics at the University of Colorado Health Sciences Center in Denver, says, "Some data suggest that women become less inhibited as they age, so it's often a time of relaxation and being comfortable with who you are, and that often improves sexual functioning and sexual performance."

Remember, when a woman no longer has to worry about getting pregnant, and her kids are probably older, she feels free to be herself. Women in this period of their lives can begin to engage in more freely open sexual encounters and welcome the opportunity to experience orgasm in a variety of newly discovered ways.

Yet, the myth of women telling their partners, "Not tonight, dear," persists, and there are many reasons for it—as well as why female desire might decline. We'll look at this more in depth later in the chapter.

In a study done by the University of California at San Diego School of Medicine, one in five sexually active women over the age of fifty reported high sexual desire. Approximately half of the women aged eighty years or more reported that they were able to become aroused and achieve climax "most of the time." Furthermore, they found that the percentage of sexually satisfied women actually increased with age, with about half of the women over eighty years old reporting sexual satisfaction "almost always" or "always."

Not only were the oldest women in this study the most satisfied overall, but they were also the ones who experienced orgasm satisfaction rates in their recent sexual activities similar to those of the youngest participants.

One of the main culprits that affects desire in women is whether they still have their ovaries. A woman who's done having babies may decide to have a hysterectomy if she's suffering from endometriosis or other uterine conditions that are negatively affecting her quality of life. If she's had her ovaries removed as well (which is called an oophorectomy and means that she will no longer produce estrogens, androgens, and progestins), she'll go into menopause and experience all the symptoms associated with it. According to Marianne Brandon, Ph.D., and Andrew Goldstein, M.D., authors of *Reclaiming Desire: 4 Keys to Finding Your Lost Libido*, not all women who have an oophorectomy experience reduced libido, so a hysterectomy doesn't necessarily spell the end of a woman's sexuality.

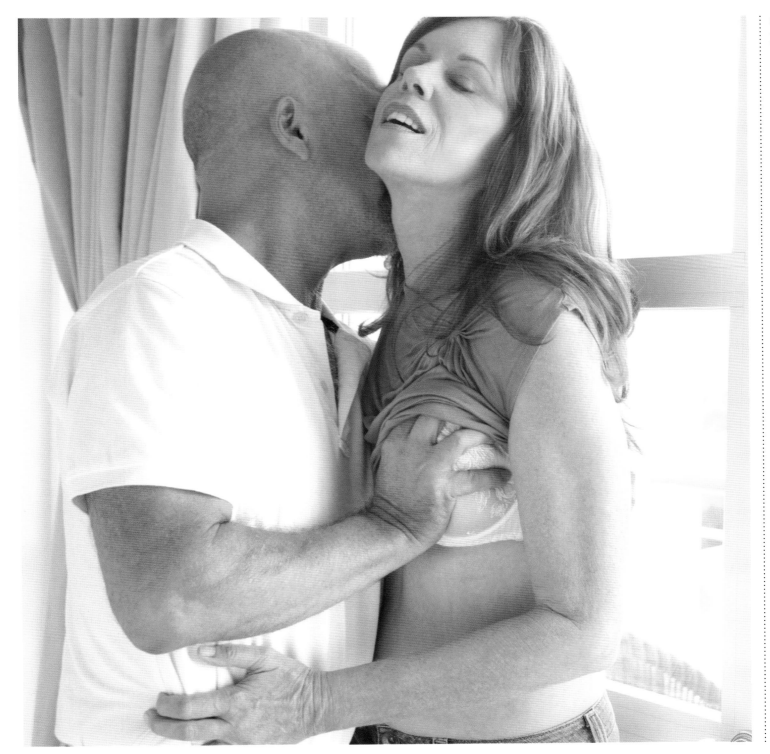

MALE DESIRE AFTER FIFTY

Generally speaking, men seem to maintain their sexual desire throughout their lives. If he had a high drive when he was a young man, he'll likely still have it later in life. However, it's certainly not uncommon for men over fifty to have a lower libido than when they were younger—just not drastically so.

Many men will tell you that they just don't feel the need for sex as much as they used to. Their interest in sex hasn't waned, but their spontaneous desire—their general "horniness"—has. This isn't something to worry about it. And women, please don't take it personally. Rarely does it have to do with you!

However, some men lose both their interest *and* their libido as they pass fifty. They notice a drastic change and are quite distressed by it. If this is the case, he should consult his doctor to determine whether there's a physical cause, such as low testosterone, side effects of a medication, depression, or some other underlying illness. By the way, in our culture, we view men as always open to sexual activity. This can put a lot of pressure on men who don't feel this way, which I'll address later in the chapter.

According to sex researcher Barry McCarthy, Ph.D., coauthor of *Rekindling Desire*, low desire affects about 15 percent of men. If he doesn't want to have sex, chances are that it isn't about his partner. Instead, he could have any of the following issues, especially if he's over fifty:
• His testosterone levels are low.
• He's depressed.
• He's stressed and/or anxious.
• He's afraid of erectile dysfunction ("performance anxiety").
• He has an underlying medical condition.
• He's taking medications that interfere with libido and sexual response (such as antidepressants, antihypertensives, and cholesterol-lowering drugs).

CASE STUDY: JIM

Jim, sixty-two, came to see me without telling his wife. He described having erectile dysfunction as well as very little interest in sex in general. "I don't want sex," he told me. "My wife brings it up every few months, and I just try to avoid that conversation at all costs. I feel completely confused, ashamed, and guilt ridden, and very much less of a man. How do I fix this?"

As a first step, I suggested he get some medical tests. It turned out that his erectile dysfunction was a side effect of his blood pressure medication. When he was unable to satisfy his wife with an erection, the thought of sex would cause him performance anxiety, and this in turn shut down his desire for sex.

Once we had the proper diagnosis, I encouraged him to bring his wife in to therapy. With them as a couple, we dealt with this new reality of sexual dysfunction, explored the treatment options—in Jim's case, his doctor prescribed him Viagra—and how to use them properly, and discussed the pressures and anxiety they were both experiencing. Once they understood the physical and psychological aspects of ED, they were well on their way to a renewed sex life together.

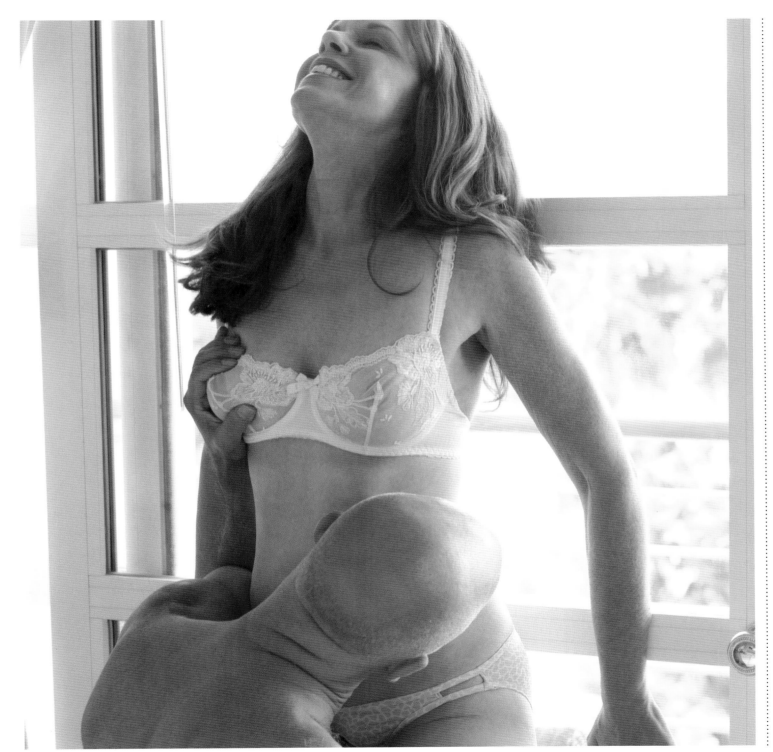

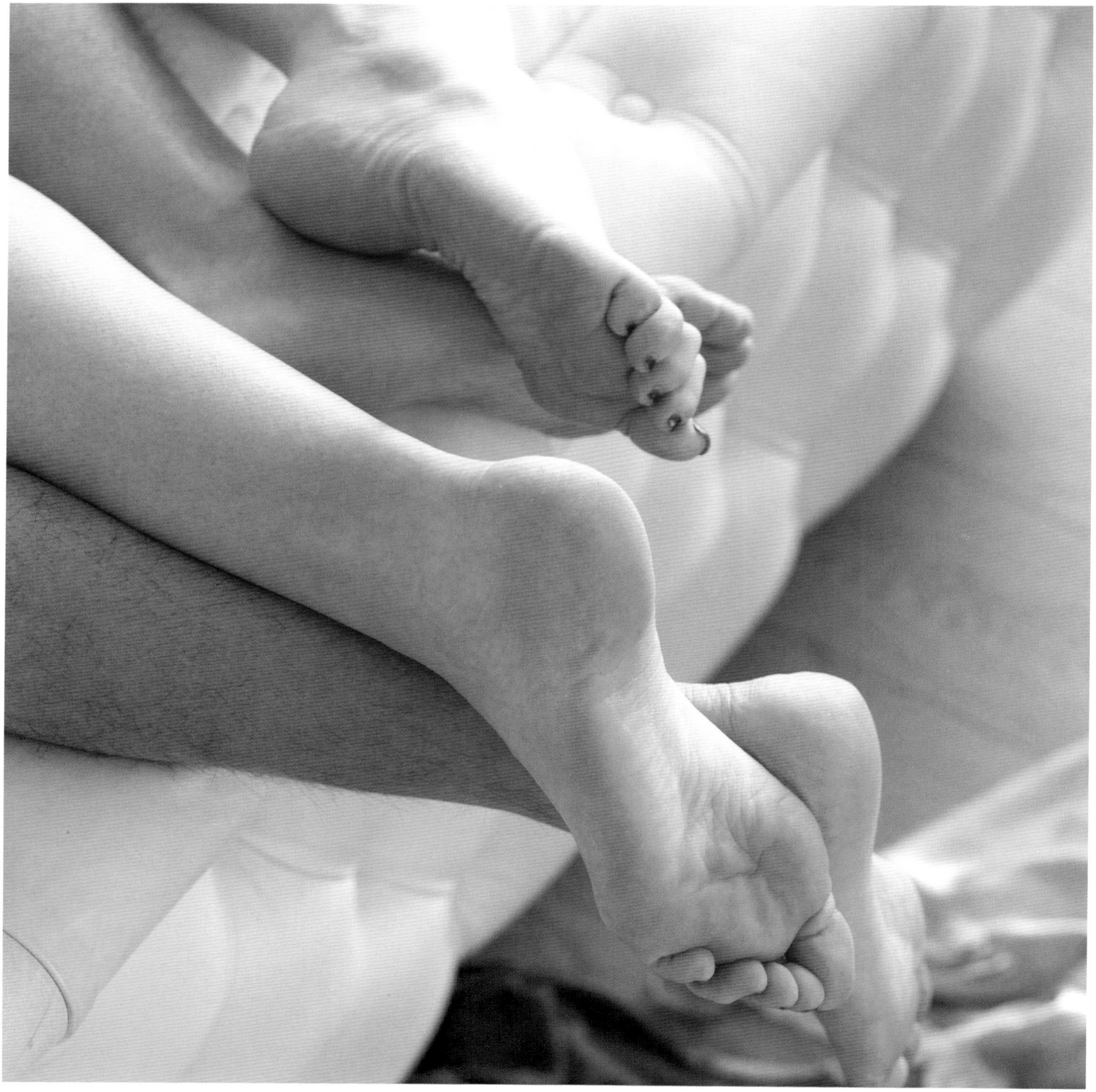

MEN VERSUS WOMEN: WHAT TRIGGERS DESIRE?

Not too long ago, we thought sexual desire looked exactly the same in men and women. Today, thanks to the work of modern sex researchers, we know differently. If most women don't experience their desire as men do, does that make them "dysfunctional"? Clearly not. So, as a first step, we need to understand these gender differences.

Here's a metaphor that sums up the way desire works for the majority of men and women in long-term relationships. Think of a car. Men are normally in "drive," and releasing the brake gets them moving. They don't even have to press on the gas pedal. Women are in "neutral" (even though many think their batteries are dead). They need an action of some sort to get them into gear. That action is a combination of physiological and psychological factors—both stimulation and context.

Let's talk a bit about the reasons men and women have sex. Generally speaking, men have sex primarily for physical pleasure, and then for intimacy. But studies show that pleasure tops the list. You may have heard the old adage that "men have sex to express love, and women need love to have sex." I've heard it myself many times over the years, but I've also seen the reverse. I've worked with many men who've told me that the older they get, the more they crave intimacy over pleasure.

Most women, on the other hand, tend to have different reasons for having sex. Not that they don't want physical pleasure, but it isn't necessarily at the top of the list. Instead, many women describe being motivated by the need to feel close to their partner, and by the positive emotional and physical experiences that they share.

According to Rosemary Basson, M.D., a psychiatrist and sex researcher in Vancouver who has written extensively on the subject of desire, what many women express as sexual needs occurs outside the bedroom. These needs include a loving emotional climate in the home, and their partner's consideration and respect, affection, and nonsexual intimacy. Sex becomes the continuation of this nonsexual intimacy; without it, women often feel like sex is a chore.

However, as women get older, many start focusing more on pleasure than on intimacy—the exact opposite of men.

DR. LAURIE'S FOUR-POINT DESIRE PLAN

This plan is a way to ease into having sex again after a long dry spell. Very important: For the first month of this plan, do NOT attempt intercourse.

Stage 1: Set aside time to spend at least 15 minutes together every day and make attempts at "romantic" gestures. If you're not sure what your partner considers romantic, ask him or her to make a list for you.

Stage 2: Kiss. Not just a peck. Start with a kiss that lasts a couple of seconds, and increase the time you lock lips each time. The goal is to get you to "make out."

Stage 3: Touch. Begin with caressing the hands, then other nonsexual body parts, with clothes on. Include cuddling and kissing.

Stage 4: Engage in sensual massage or naked touching. Start with caressing naked nonsexual parts, and move to touching genitals.

If you follow this plan for one month, and neither of you feels pressured, you can start having sexual intercourse. Some couples really enjoy these stages and want to spend more time on them, and actually choose to hold off!

Three Levels of Female Desire

Michael Krychman, M.D., says in his book *100 Questions & Answers About Women's Sexual Wellness and Vitality: A Practical Guide for the Woman Seeking Sexual Fulfillment* that women fall into three general categories with respect to desire and sexual response:

• *Low to moderate desire.* For about one-third of women, sexual desire escalates or diminishes depending on context. For example, if the kids are awake, she can't relax for fear she and her partner will be heard. Her desire is there, but the context has to be right.

• *Sexually neutral.* Another third of women respond to cues from their partner or their environment. She might get the warm-and-fuzzies because her partner did something special, for example. Without these feelings, she feels neutral about sex. She can go without it and not really miss it. It's the warmth she feels toward her partner that will make her "open" to sex.

• *Pursuers.* The remaining third of women have a hunger and strong desire for sex. Three-fourths of men fall into this category, by the way, which scientists believe is mostly due to biology rather than culture.

An example I often use to illustrate the difference between men and women's desire is this: A woman walks out of the shower naked; her partner takes a look at her and is likely to get aroused, erection and all. Now let's reverse this little scenario. He walks out of the shower naked. Does her clitoris suddenly begin to throb, in the equivalent of an erection? If she's lucky it might, but chances are it will take more than the sight of his nakedness to trigger desire in her.

Female sexual desire is affected by myriad factors that include stress, fatigue, anger, resentment, hormones, dishes in the sink, socks on the floor, etc. It's almost as if most women have a hard time shutting out the world to just focus on their bodies. As women age, I have found that many learn to care less about the little things and they start to focus more on their own needs and wants, often prioritizing pleasure in all of its forms. This results in more *decisions* to allow herself the sexual pleasure with her partner, which in turn will trigger more of the desire. She may never be triggered in the same way her mate is, but that doesn't mean she isn't *interested* in sex.

That's not to say that a man's desire isn't affected in similar ways. Men just seem to be better at shutting off the main valve to allow their desires to flow. I don't mean to imply that men never suffer from low sexual desire. They certainly do, and the factors that affect them are similar to those affecting women with low desire.

STRATEGIES FOR IGNITING DESIRE

Men, as we've seen, don't generally have an issue with desire (although it happens—see page 77). So when it comes to strategies for igniting that craving in women, it falls on both partners.

Women need to understand that they can't just wait for that "horny" feeling to magically appear before they engage in sex. We now know that women have to be sexually stimulated before they feel desire. For many women, once they allow themselves to be stimulated—by hand, mouth, vibrator, or whatever—get physically aroused and their desire kicks in. But before a woman can allow herself to be stimulated, her partner first needs to satisfy her conditions.

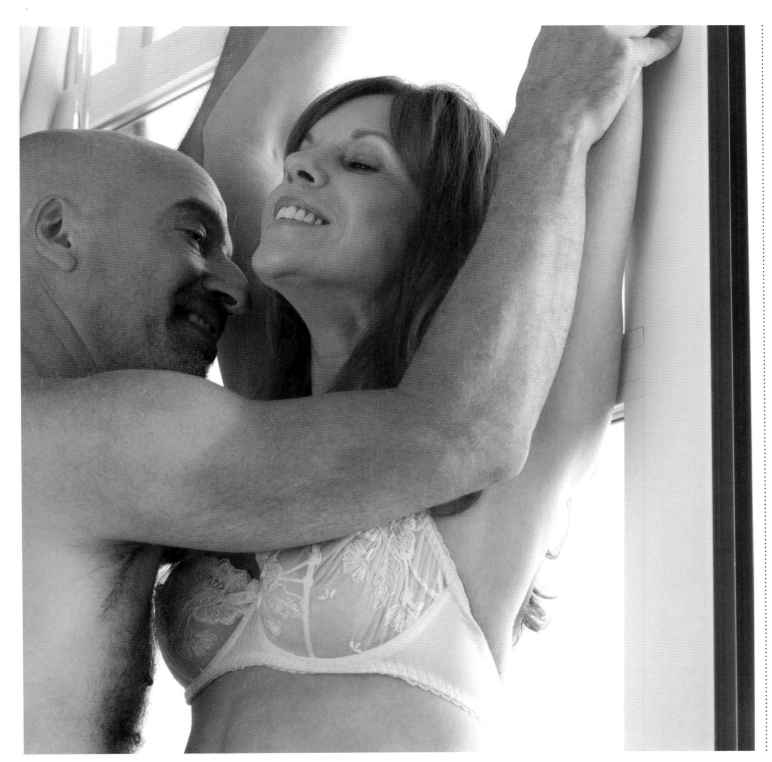

Men often roll their eyes when I start talking about their partner needing certain conditions to be met before she even considers having sex. But once he understands what she needs outside of the bedroom, he gets to reap the benefits *in* the bedroom. Here are a few guidelines:

• First and foremost, don't pressure her for sex (even subtly).

• Show her affection and romance without expecting it to go further.

• Show her that you love her for her, and not the sex she can give you.

• Don't make her feel that she's responsible for your erection.

• Ask her what she needs from you to alleviate her own stress (even if that means cleaning the toilets), and then do it.

If you do this, the chances are good that she'll start to feel warmly toward you, and this will lead to her being more open to having sex.

GETTING FROM POINT A TO POINT B

Usually, once a woman makes the decision to have sex and allows herself to become aroused, her desire is triggered and she'll want to continue sexual activity. Yet many women tell me that the major issue they have is getting from point A to point B. They know they should have sex, they know they enjoy sex when they do it, they rarely regret doing it, and they feel really good after they do it. So why don't they just DO IT?

For the same reason they don't go to the gym as often as they know they should. They know the gym is good for them, they feel good when they've worked out, and they enjoy working out when they're there. But the hard part is waking up at 5 a.m. to get their butts there. See a parallel? Inertia takes over, and before you know it, years have passed. (This is true for both sex and the gym.) The key is to change your mind-set and make sex (and the gym) a part of your lifestyle and your routine.

To get over your inertia, give the Sex Strategies outlined in this chapter a whirl.

WHAT ABOUT IGNITING *HIS* DESIRE?

Male desire isn't always a sure thing. When it seems as if it's more "off" than "on," the first step is to look for the underlying cause of his low desire. Is it psychological or physical? Next, take the pressure off the need to have an erection. Men can be sexual without one. It's a good time to explore different ways to pleasure your partner, and let her make you feel good without trying to get you hard. Focus more on total body pleasure and creating intimacy between the two of you. As you feel closer and less pressured to "perform," your desire for sexuality will be triggered.

SEX STRATEGY: HE DECIDES THE "WHEN," SHE DECIDES THE "HOW"

This is a strategy I adopted from Pat Love, Ed.D., who gives wonderful workshops on keeping passion alive. Use this only if there aren't any major relationship issues at the root of the low desire, and both of you still feel sexual interest and arousal.

He gets to ask for sex anytime.

She decides whether it will be a "quickie," oral sex, manual sex, or any other form of sex.

The result: He tends to ask for sex less because he knows he can get it anytime, and she feels more in control of the sexuality, which makes her feel less pressured.

GETTING OUT OF THE RUT

According to some estimates, one in four relationships are considered sexless. In other words, the couple has sex only a few times a year, or not at all. I see many couples that have ended up in this situation without a clue as to how they got there. It just seemed to "happen."

Once they decide to do something about rediscovering their sexuality as a couple, they often describe feeling awkward about it again. THIS IS NORMAL. But it's like riding a bike again. You may be a little shaky at first, but with a little practice, it will all come back to you. It really is okay to laugh at yourselves, and men, it's certainly okay if you don't get an erection the first few times. Know that your early attempts may be awkward, and find the humor in it. You're working toward the same goal—more and better sex.

STRATEGIES TO BOOST DESIRE (ONCE IT'S REIGNITED)

Now that you've lit the flame of desire, how can you fan it into a raging fire? As we accumulate birthdays, we need more to get us going. We need more direct, more intense touch—and we need more to stimulate arousal, which, after all, begins in the brain. Here are a few ideas.

Get Rid of Distractions

Sometimes life gets stressful. Those over fifty often find themselves in the "sandwich generation," with demands coming from their kids and from their aging parents. Not to mention the fact that no one retires young anymore! So we need to make time for the fun stuff—such as sex.

Think about what you need to do to empty your mind of your troubles, just for a short time. Most couples describe "vacation sex" as pretty great. Why? No distractions. So you may need to take mini-vacations, even in your own city. Every once in a while, book yourselves into a hotel room and let someone else take care of making the bed in the morning.

Talk Dirty

Stimulating the mind is a huge part of desire and attraction. What better way to do it than by voicing your erotic thoughts? Being more vocal during sex, especially during foreplay, can help you and your partner achieve a more intense level of sexual experience. What you say is completely up to you. It may turn you both on to use crude or explicit language to describe what you like or what you're feeling: "I want to fuck you," "I love your big, hard, cock"—you get the idea.

Of course, if you and your partner have never talked dirty to each other before, don't jump right in with the most naughty requests and comments you can think of. It might take your partner completely off guard. Start slow.

On the other hand, if you and your partner already engage in dirty talk regularly, kick it up a notch. Talk about things you might want to try, or consider sharing your fantasies with one another.

CASE STUDY: ADAM AND OLIVIA

Olivia, fifty-two, came to see me alone, saying that her husband, Adam, fifty-one, was very frustrated because she just didn't feel like having sex as much as he did. He told her there was something wrong with her, and he wanted her to "get checked out." He was convinced she had a physical condition. She was convinced she wasn't normal.

Olivia said she enjoyed sex when they had it, she occasionally masturbated, and she loved reading steamy novels. We concluded that her interest in sex was intact.

Was he the problem? Olivia felt Adam was constantly "after her" for sex. She felt pressured, and complained that he only touched her intimately in hopes that it would lead to sex.

Then they visited me as a couple. Aside from the sexual issue, both described a loving, strong relationship. Both got a lesson on the facts about desire for men and women. We explored what Olivia needed to feel open to sex. They went home with Dr. Laurie's Four-Point Desire Plan (see sidebar on page 73) and did their "homework."

Olivia reports that she loves not being pressured and is much more open to sex because she's feeling much closer to Adam. Adam, for his part, finds it a bit difficult to "hold back," but he recognizes the great benefit in doing so!

Talking dirty doesn't necessarily mean face-to-face conversation. You could send a descriptive email or naughty text message ("sexting"), or leave a note in his or her briefcase or gym bag. This will have your partner thinking about sex all day. It's another form of foreplay!

Write Your Own Erotica
Both men and women fantasize, with the main gender difference being the content of fantasies. Women tend to have more romantic fantasies; men, more explicit ones. Fantasies can induce or enhance sexual arousal. They also serve as a form of rehearsal for practicing things you might want to try in real life.

Interestingly, sexual fantasies don't seem to change with age; however, we are likelier to have experienced more variety of sexual activity, which in turn can fuel our fantasies. So it stands to reason that the older we are, the more varied our fantasies may become. Here's a simple formula for exploring your own fantasies—by crafting your own erotica.

• Make a list of erotic thoughts or ideas that turn you on (such as having a threesome).
• Make a list of your exotic, erotic places—a beach, a limo, a restaurant bathroom.
• Involve your senses. Think of some erotic sensations, such as the feel of satin sheets, the smell of a scented candle, or the feel of latex.
• Write down a fantasy plot. Maybe your heroine gets seduced—or does the seducing.
• List the traits of your main characters, including their appearance and even their occupation (hunky firefighter, red-haired dominatrix).
• Read steamy novels and note the scenes that turn you on the most. If you prefer visuals, think of an experience you once had that was really hot, or draw from a story in porn. Practice visualizing the scene while in a state of relaxation.
• Now construct your own fantasy scene. First close your eyes and relax. Think of an erotic scenario, and imagine all the small details (the where, the how, and all the physical sensations you feel). Focus most on the erotic details, such as the feel of the other person's body. Then practice recalling the scenario. Practice, practice!
• You can also write down your entire sexual fantasy on paper instead of just recalling it to mind.

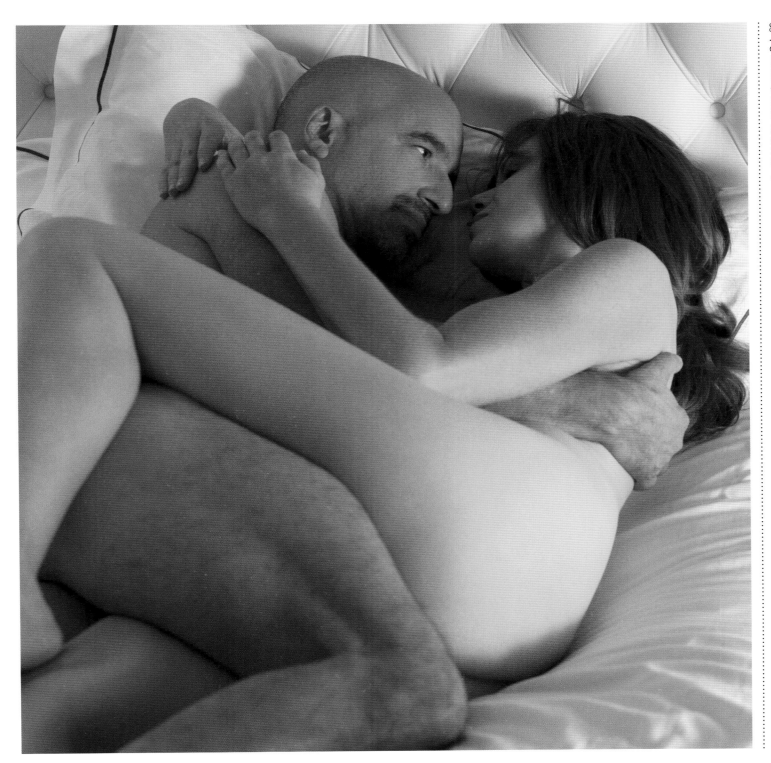

CASE STUDY: ALEXIA AND CHARLIE

Alexia and Charlie, in their late forties and married for fifteen years, regularly role-play a scenario in which they pretend to have just met. Alexia leaves the house first and agrees to meet Charlie at a specific bar. She sits at the bar by herself. A little while later, Charlie walks in and "makes the moves" on Alexia as if he's a stranger who's just spotted a beautiful girl he wants to take home. Sometimes it's Alexia who does the seducing. This has made a huge difference in their sex life!

Stimulate Your Brain

Watching or looking at pornography together as a couple can do wonders to ignite sexual arousal. Pick a film that has some sort of storyline, as this tends to be more stimulating for women; porn made by female directors/producers often offer decent plots. (A great place to look for such movies is www.goodforher.com.) What's more, choosing porn together will also get you talking about what you would like to see. It's another way to feed those fantasies you're creating in your mind.

Thanks to television shows like *Sex in the City* and books like *50 Shades of Grey*, women today are much less secretive about their interest in sex. As a result, there's been a proliferation of erotic writing geared toward women over the past few years. It's certainly not unusual to see a woman reading an erotic novel, even on a public bus. So try reading a story aloud to each other!

Get Some Distance (for a Night)

Remember those days when you were first dating and getting to know each other? Remember how hot the sex was at the beginning? Mystery about our partner fuels desire. As Esther Perel, a marriage and family therapist and author of *Mating in Captivity: Unlocking Erotic Intelligence*, says, "Love seeks closeness, desire needs distance." Try this exercise: Look at your partner as someone outside your relationship would see him or her. Or try role-playing a scenario in which you go to a bar separately and seduce each other. It will most definitely end in you taking each other home for some action!

Masturbate for Better Partner Sex

Self-pleasure is always a good thing, but it's even more important as you get older and your body begins to change. For one thing, it keeps your blood flowing, which keeps your genitals healthy, which in turn leads to better sex. Second, it allows you to figure out how you need to be touched so that you can show or communicate this to your partner. Third, it gets you feeling aroused, which can prepare you for—and get you interested in—partner sex.

Set aside some uninterrupted time for yourself. Do something relaxing such as taking a bath or performing some meditation exercises. Pull out your favorite sex toy (see more on sex toys in chapter 8) and/or lubricant, and just focus on bodily sensations. Orgasm isn't the goal. Arousal is.

The Affection Connection

Sex feels great. But the reality is that we don't have sex for hours every day, so it's important to stay physically connected in other ways so that we can stay in that after-sex glow for as long as possible. I'm talking about nonsexual touch. Don't forget or get too busy to connect physically throughout the day, whether it's with a light caress, a hug, a kiss, or a pat on the behind. Any gesture that says "I love you" keeps you and your partner connected.

DESIRE BUSTERS—AND WHAT TO DO ABOUT THEM

For some men and women, hormones play a big role in desire. For others, a negative belief system, relationship issues, or stress affect their levels of desire. Let's take a closer look.

Stress

Stress is the number-one desire killer for both sexes. Stress means we're worried about all kinds of things, and worry is a state of mind that impedes relaxation. When our minds are full of worries, sex is definitely not on our brains; this seems truer for women than for men. We need to learn how to manage stress so it doesn't stop us from enjoying one of life's greatest pleasures (sex!).

Unfortunately, most of us can't escape the realities of life as an older adult—dealing with teenaged kids or paying for college, work (or loss of), taking care of aging parents, etc. However, our attitudes toward these situations determines how stressed we feel. The paradox, of course, is that sex can be a great stress buster!

Stress-reducing strategies: Take care of your physical self by exercising. Take care of your psychological self by "letting go" of the things you can't control. Take care of some of your responsibilities by delegating. Take care of your relationship by having at least one "date night" a week.

Hormones

Testosterone is the dominant hormone when it comes to sex drive; a shortage of it can result in reduced sexual desire. Both men and women produce testosterone, though women produce much smaller amounts. Testosterone levels peak in both genders in the early to mid-twenties and then begin a steady decline.

For men, testosterone production continues throughout their lifetime. As I discussed in chapter 4, some men may experience testosterone deficiency syndrome as they grow older, and this will have an impact on their sexuality. The same can happen for women as they produce much less estrogens and androgens, which are also responsible, in part, for sexual feelings.

Emotional Intimacy

Feeling close to your partner plays a major part in increasing desire, especially for women. If you and your partner are suffering from poor communication or trust issues, address those with a therapist first before you focus on your sex life. If all seems good, yet you feel like you are living with your roommate, you need to start addressing the elephant in the room. It's perfectly normal to feel awkward at first, especially if it's been a while, so try to have some fun with this. Plan on just hanging out naked in bed, massage each other, play strip poker . . . as long as it's fun and you can laugh about it.

Sleep

An issue that accompanies us as we age is disturbed sleep. Whether it's hot flashes, sleep apnea, or aches and pains that keep us awake at night, too little sleep will sap anyone of sexy feelings.

Medications

Many common medications—certain antidepressants, blood pressure medications, sedatives, and cholesterol medications—can hamper drive and arousal. Doctors are often remiss in discussing the potential sexual side effects of medications, so don't be embarrassed to ask! Tell your doctor if your sex drive seems affected soon after you start taking a new medication.

Depression

Low sexual desire can sometimes be a symptom of depression. Unfortunately, antidepressants can further decrease desire as well as the ability to orgasm. However, depression can be potentially life-threatening, so if you've been feeling sad, hopeless, irritable, anxious, empty, and unmotivated, and feel like you no longer take pleasure in many things you used to enjoy, then please see your doctor. Some newer antidepressants—as well as older ones like Wellbutrin—have fewer sexual side effects.

According to the National Institute of Mental Health, only 1 to 2 percent of people over age sixty-five who live independently suffer from diagnosed major depression. An additional 13 to 27 percent of older adults have subclinical depression that, although it doesn't fit the criteria for major depression, is associated with an increased risk of it, as well as physical disability, medical illness, and high use of health services.

Alcohol Use

Chronic use of alcohol has been shown to affect hormone levels and cause other medical problems that play a role in sexuality. Alcohol dependency can result in sexual problems that include low libido, premature ejaculation, erectile dysfunction, and difficulty achieving orgasm. These problems may be caused by the depressant effect of alcohol itself, alcohol-related diseases, or the multitude of psychological issues related to the alcohol use. If you think you or your partner might suffer from alcoholism (and there are numerous online quizzes to help you determine that), please seek help. Even if your alcohol use is moderate, please note that although one or two drinks will relax you and might get you in the mood for sex, more than that can cause some of the problems outlined here.

Body Image

Feeling sexy is a whole lot easier if we like how we look in the mirror. Body image issues can certainly put a damper on our sex lives if we don't learn to accept our bodies as they are *today*. Feeling good about yourself will help bring the sexy back! While we can't fight the effects of time, we can slow its march with a positive, accepting attitude. Maybe a new haircut or color is in order. Perhaps a closet purge will do the trick. Though your twenty-something self might seem like a distant memory, it doesn't mean that you can't look the best you've ever looked *right now*.

If the Spirit Is Willing …

If you're experiencing a decline in sexual desire, don't ignore it. Address the issues that got you there, and gain an understanding of how your libido can be affected by your life circumstances. Also know that when the spirit is willing, the body will follow—with the help of the right strategies.

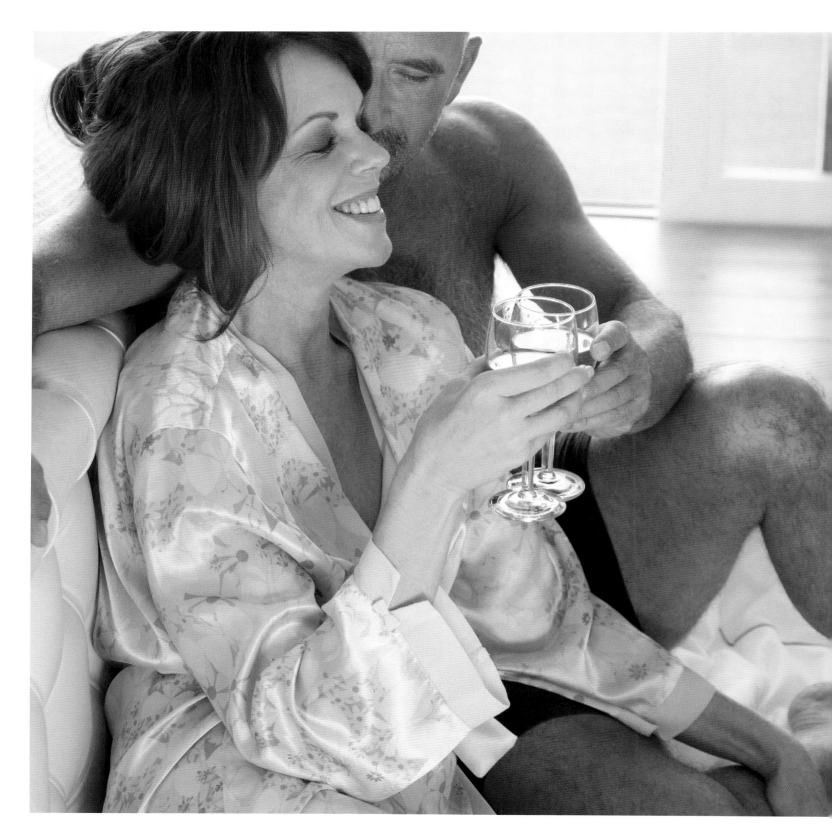

06 *Setting the Stage for Seduction*

One of the by-products of our busy lives is just that: We're busy. Whether it's endless meetings and business trips; running between swim meets, basketball games, and college interviews; or taking Mom and Dad to doctor appointments between shoveling their snow and buying their groceries, it's a wonder we have any time for ourselves, let alone our partners.

It's little surprise, then, that a common complaint I hear from couples is that they just can't get in the mood. With our hectic lifestyles, it's hard to change gears at the end of the day to get into a more relaxed, sensual state of mind.

We need to take charge of this "not in the mood" situation and do something about it. That means we have to consciously work to overcome the crazy pace of our lives and set a more sexual mood. I'm not talking big changes here. There are small changes that you can start making right away.

"Setting the mood," however, isn't something you do for only one night. Devote some time every day to making your life and your environment more sensual. By doing so, you'll generate a more sexual mood in your daily life.

CREATING YOUR LOVE NEST

Take a look at your bedroom. Does it look exactly the same as the day you moved in thirty years ago? Ask yourself: Does this room make me feel sexy? Does this room make me feel romantic? If your answer is "no," then your first step is to make some changes to the decor to give it a more romantic, sensual ambience. Improving the environment in your boudoir can go a long way toward spicing up what happens in it.

To make your bedroom more romantic, concentrate on creating a relaxing haven that pleases all of the senses. Talk with your partner about the kinds of things that make you feel sexy. Incorporate those things into your bedroom.

Specifically, use different textures on your bed. For example, pair crisp sheets with a satin or velvet blanket and big soft pillows. This will help create a welcoming and cozy place to hang out. Hang richly textured curtains rather than venetian blinds. Choose colors in warm tones. Fill your room with different scents, and change them with the seasons. Go for richer, warmer scents such as vanilla in winter, and try fresher fragrances in spring. Avoid stark, super-bright overhead lights. Install bulbs with lower wattages or pink-toned hues, as they provide more flattering lighting. Or turn off the lights and use candles. Keep a small sound system in your room along with your favorite CDs, or make a sexy playlist for your iPod. And if the rest of your living space will allow for it, remove any exercise equipment from your bedroom—especially if it tends to collect more laundry than burnt calories. Ditto for the television. It's difficult to become romantic with the nightly news or late-night comedy on the tube, so remove it or turn it off. Your bedroom should be for sleeping and intimacy.

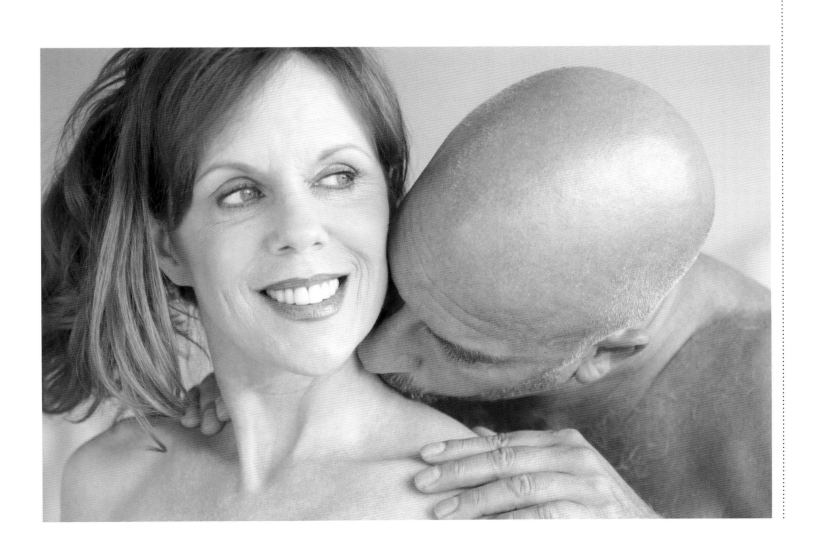

THE FRANK KERMIT
ROMANCE FORMULA

My good friend and colleague Frank Kermit, a relationship expert and former "seduction" coach, has developed a sure-fire formula for creating the ultimate context for sex. He says it's a tried-and-true approach; he's seen many people use with success. Here it is:

1. Stimulate the five senses. For instance:
• Sight: Light some candles, wear a beautiful negligee.
• Sound: Play soft music.
• Taste: Serve sexy appetizers, such as caviar and fresh fruit, and pair them with a bottle of wine.
• Smell: Place fragrant flowers in the room or wear your partner's favorite perfume or aftershave.

2. Touch: Massage your partner's shoulders:
• Address the emotional needs of your partner.
• She needs to feel desired for more than just sex.
• He may need to feel fully appreciated for his efforts.

3. Incorporate sensual or sexual context when you're together:
• Throughout the romantic encounter, allude to the sex you're going to have later through teasing, playful words, and gestures.

It's definitely important to appeal to the five senses; however, even more important is addressing your partner's unique emotional needs. Think about what he or she would best respond to. For example, she may need to feel fully accepted for the noises she makes during sex, and he may need to feel fully appreciated for providing for his family.

In this time when we're surrounded by so many electronic devices, it's crucial that you communicate to your partner through words and gestures that you're going to focus on just the two of you. The goal of romance is to set the stage for a sexual encounter. Create anticipation by alluding to the upcoming sexual experience before you even get into the bedroom by touching her in a sensual way, or telling him how you're looking forward to undressing him!

PLAN, PLAN, PLAN

For some reason, many of us believe that the best sex has to be spontaneous. But those of us who have kids and other distractions know that if we wait for spontaneity to happen, we'd rarely have sex. Planning for sex is what keeps us focused on the relationship.

So how do we do this, if our teenage kids stay up way past our bedtime? How do we get past the fear that they will hear us doing the deed? Try, for example, installing a lock on your bedroom door if your kids have a tendency to just barge in. Also, keep in mind that older kids are busy doing their thing, usually in their rooms with the door closed, headphones on. Not to mention that they really don't care (and don't want to know) what you're doing behind your closed door! And just think of the erotic fun you can have coming up with new positions or locations that don't require your creaky bed.

Spontaneous sex is a myth, says Barbara Hannah Grufferman, AARP columnist, show host, and author of *The Best of Everything After 50: The Experts' Guide to Style, Sex, Health, Money, and More*. She contends that sex was never spontaneous in the first place, and "good sex never is." Planning for sex can be sexy. Imagine all that anticipation of the erotic journey ahead.

There's absolutely nothing wrong with needing a little nudge to have sex. As mentioned in the previous chapter, sometimes it's like going to the gym. Once we talk ourselves into it, the outcome is usually great. Of course, as we've seen, aging can have its physical and emotional challenges, making planning that much more important (I'll discuss this more in chapter 8). Bottom line: It's okay to choose *and* plan for fun, play, and pleasure. The rest of our lives are commandeered by a calendar—why not add sex to it? And once it's there, stick to it. After all, you wouldn't cancel on your dentist or accountant, would you?

FOREPLAY AFTER FIFTY

Foreplay is important at any age. Study after study demonstrates the benefits of foreplay for increasing arousal and achieving orgasm. As we start the second half of our lives, however, it becomes even more crucial. Because it takes us longer to get aroused—longer to get an erection or to lubricate—we MUST spend time engaged in non-intercourse ("outercourse") activities. Spend at least 15 to 20 minutes hugging, holding, and kissing your partner. Take your time slowly undressing him or her. Don't rush to the end goal of getting naked. As you remove each article of clothing, use it as an opportunity to caress and touch. If you've been with your partner for many years, anticipation can wane in sex—after all, you've probably seen your partner's body thousands of times and sex can follow an all-too-predictable routine. Think back to when you first met your partner and sex wasn't a given yet—you probably had to work to seduce him or her. You may not have started your physical relationship with intercourse, but you probably spent those initial days, weeks, or even months of courtship letting kissing, touching, and making out be the ultimate. Use that strategy again. Spend time teasing each other by discussing fantasies, giving each other a massage, and then proceeding to sex. Foreplay promotes intimacy, develops trust, increases emotional connection, and deepens love, not to mention the fact that it greatly increases sexual satisfaction.

CASE STUDY: CAROLINE AND STEVE

Caroline, fifty-nine, came to see me because her husband Steve, sixty-one, was having trouble with his erections, and she wanted to know how she could help him. She said that when they had sex, it was all about intercourse. The minute he got an erection, he immediately wanted to enter her for fear of losing it. This didn't sit well with Caroline, who wasn't nearly ready for penetration.

When I met with him, I saw that he clearly understood that foreplay was important for her, but he felt caught in a catch-22. As they discussed sex more openly, it became clear to him that intercourse was not really what gave his wife pleasure. Intercourse was also not an absolute necessity for him.

The plan, therefore, was for them to engage in "outercourse" without the goal of eventual intercourse. If his erection lasted, then they could attempt intercourse, but only once Caroline was satisfied and well lubricated. They were both very happy with this plan of action and reported feeling less pressured and more relaxed during sexual activity.

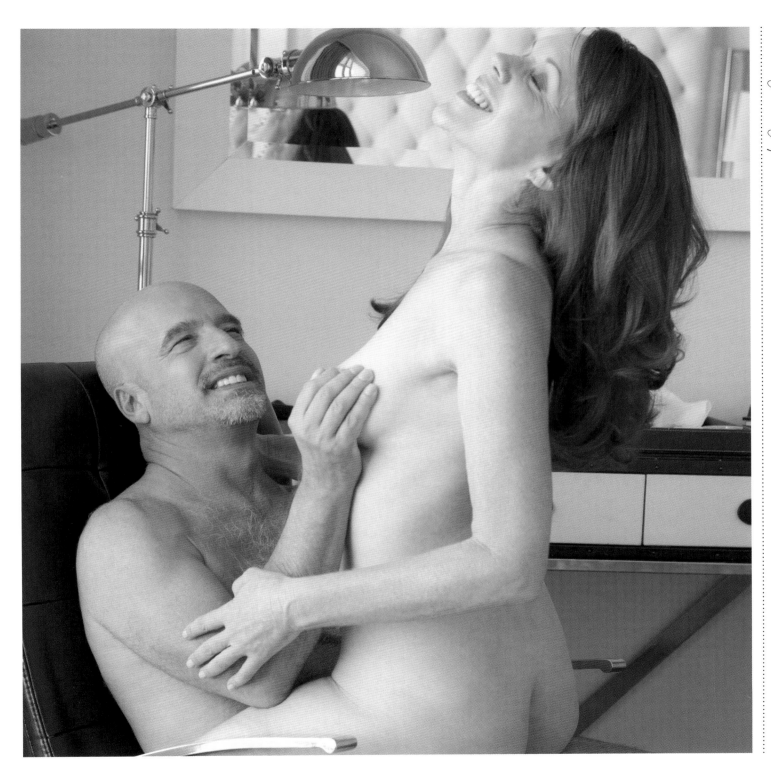

Foreplay for Him

Our sexual needs and wants change over time. Men tend to place more importance on intimacy, touch, and affection as they mature. Many say that that while intercourse is nice, it's no longer the absolute necessity it once was. It's almost as if they now can appreciate a slower pace, relishing each moment of physical connectedness.

In fact, a study conducted by the University of New Brunswick in Canada found that men ideally would like to spend 18 minutes engaged in foreplay. But women believed that men only wanted at most 13 minutes! Here are some tips and techniques a woman can use with her partner.

Use your mouth: Because it may take your man longer to achieve an erection, and he'll need more direct stimulation to get there, your mouth is the perfect way to get him aroused. By putting your mouth on his penis, you can provide a "tighter" suction than your vagina would allow. You can also use your hands at the same time to provide even more friction (see the section on oral sex in chapter 8 for more detailed techniques).

Use your hand: Use your hand to masturbate him. Try a tighter grip on his penis to provide more friction (which he will need as he gets older)—but use a lubricant or lotion. You can also ask him to show you or guide you so that you know exactly what kind of pressure to apply and what kind of movement he prefers. Don't forget to let your hands roam all over his body, including his testicles. Try cupping, then lifting, his testicles a little closer to his body.

Use your breasts: You can use your breasts as a sex toy. Try rubbing some lubricant or oil on your breasts. Have him glide up your body so that his penis is between them. You then use your hands to squeeze your breasts around his penis and move them around (or he can move back and forth, depending on how well he can hold himself in that position). You may need to find a different position, such as woman on top, if he can't hold his weight up on his arms.

Use your whole body: Mature men often describe having "whole body" orgasms. Their pleasure is no longer concentrated just on their genitals. Try a "body-body" massage. To do it, grease yourself up with oil and lie on top of him. Move your body up and down and side to side. It's extremely sensual and arousing, and gives him a very different kind of sensation.

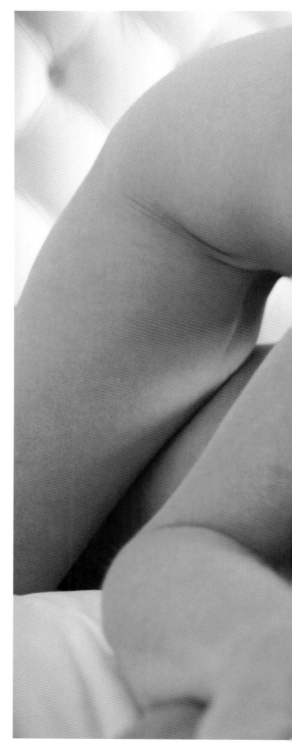

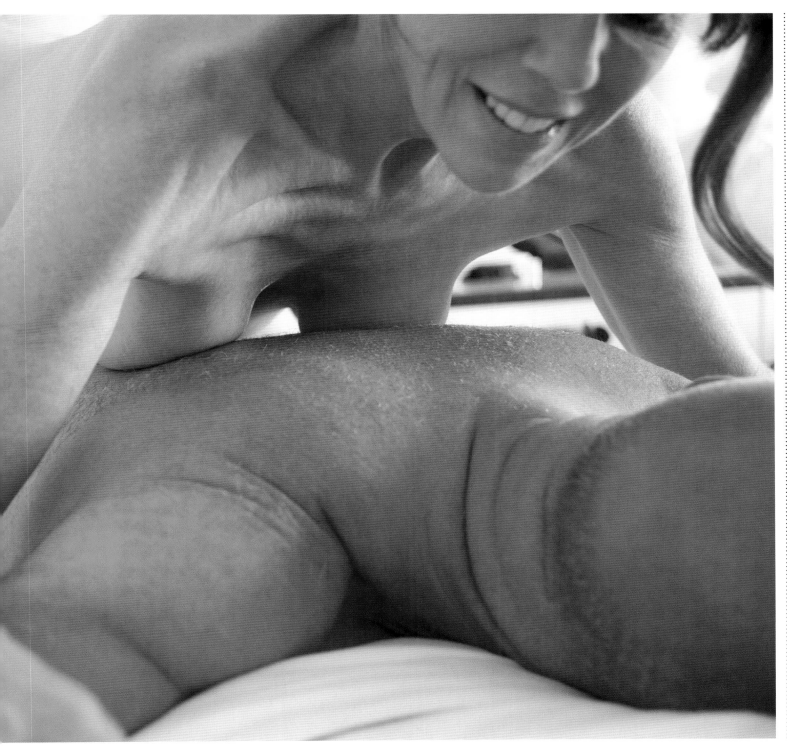

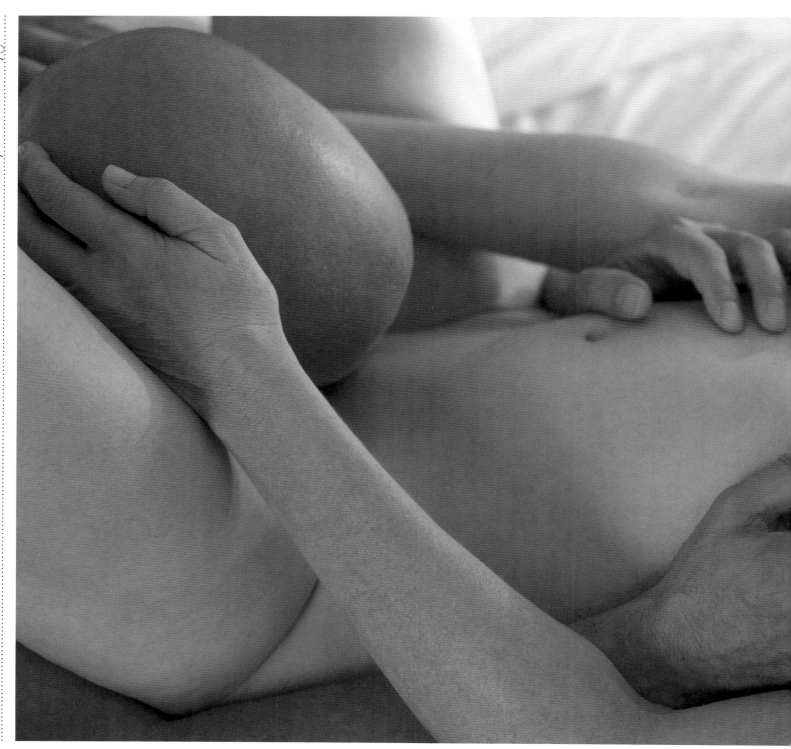

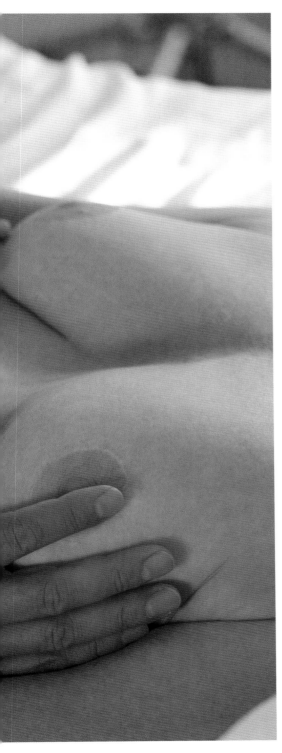

Foreplay for Her

Women need foreplay. Period. As it so happens, mature men tend to be more concerned about their partner's pleasure than their own. They're very willing to take the time to pleasure her in every which way possible. It's no fun for him if she's not enjoying herself. As she gets older, what feels good may change, so you can't necessarily rely on your old "moves." Instead, try these tips and techniques.

Use your fingers: Because her vagina may take longer to get lubricated, and her vaginal lining is thinner, it's more prone to small cuts. So keep your nails short, and lubricate your fingers either with saliva or some lubricant. If the skin on your fingers is rough, you can buy finger condoms, which are basically latex "gloves," but only for your finger. This will ensure smoothness going in.

Fingers are a great way to access her G-spot. Insert your lubricated index finger into her vagina and do a "come here" motion. This area contains very sensitive nerve endings that, when stimulated, can lead to a very intense orgasm.

Use a clitoral stimulator: As a woman ages, she may lose some sensation in her clitoris or simply require more intense stimulation. A clitoral stimulator or vibrator can be a great addition to your foreplay. First, a clitoral vibrator will do most of the work—a big advantage if you have arthritis in your hands—as all you have to do is move it around a bit. Second, the stimulation it offers is more intense than what your hand or mouth can offer.

Use your mouth (and tongue): Your tongue is very soft. Instead of your finger, try penetrating her vagina with your tongue. Use your tongue on her clitoris, and maybe provide a little suction action. Always pay attention to whether she is enjoying this or not. If in doubt, ask! Use your mouth all over her body. Kiss her everywhere. This will send her the message that her body arouses you, no matter its age.

FOREPLAY? MORE PLAY!

With age, both partners will need a little extra spice to get fully aroused and achieve maximum pleasure. It's important to communicate to your partner, verbally or by showing, what you need and want. Do you want to be caressed harder, kissed more lightly, rubbed faster or slower? This needs to be communicated, and foreplay is the perfect time to learn what your partner likes.

Remember that you can never spend too much time on foreplay. It can only enhance the sexual encounter and the relationship.

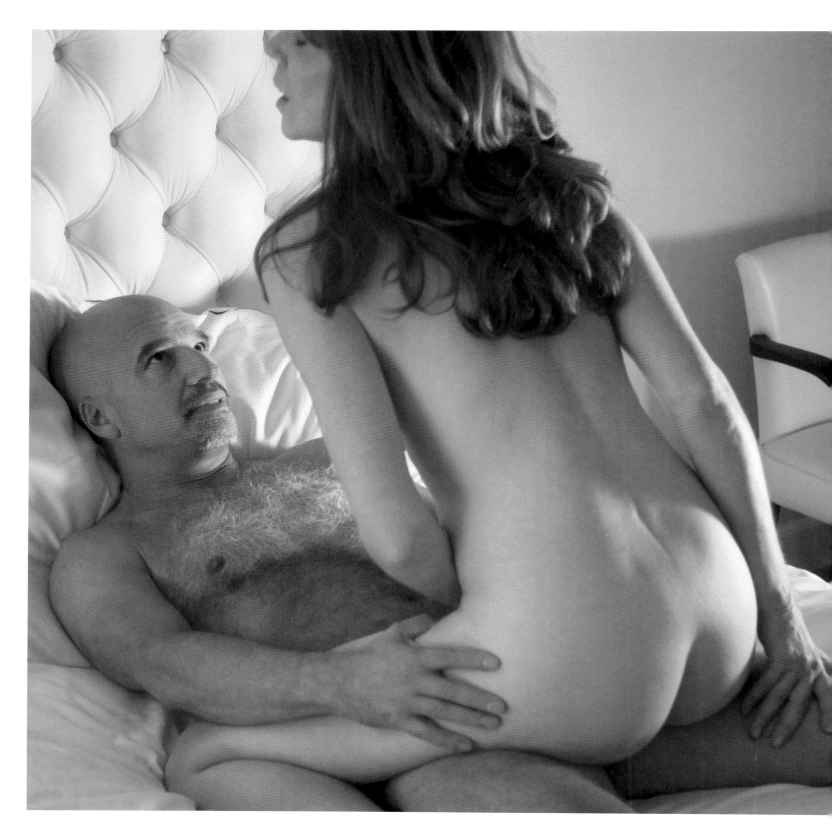

♂♀ 07 Easy Kama Sutra after Fifty

James, fifty-three, came to see me about three months after having a knee replacement. He told me that since the operation, he'd been avoiding sex for fear that it would hurt and he'd damage his knee again. Shirley, his fifty-one-year-old wife, was very understanding and urged him to get help, because she was noticing that this was also affecting his moods and how he felt about himself.

It turns out that he and his wife had been having intercourse the same way for thirty years: missionary style, with him on top—which, of course, put pressure on his knees!

The first step for them was to communicate their fears to each other and discuss sex openly so that they could explore different ways of being sexual instead of avoiding sex altogether. It was wonderful to see how they opened up to each other about sexuality. They were able to resolve their issues by trying new techniques and positions. I'm telling you this story to re-emphasize that sex doesn't have to end once you pass fifty, even if you have chronic health conditions!

Getting older doesn't necessarily mean getting out of shape. It means that you may be able to move your body in all kinds of ways without impediment or pain, so there's no reason you can't try just about any position your body allows. On the other hand, it's perfectly normal if, as we mature, our bodies don't hold up as well as our minds. In our *heads* we're still able to tackle any position, but the reality can be painful or uncomfortable.

Nonetheless, it's still possible to have a great sex life! It's still possible to get into unique positions. It's still possible to make sex adventurous. You just can't expect to approach sex in the same way you did in your teens or early twenties. Exciting sex is still on the table; it's just that the menu has a few nuances.

You can still get the aspects of what you liked in a position you enjoyed previously. You just need to find ways to support your body where needed, and stay clear of activities that would directly challenge your well-being. With a little education and some hot sex tips, you can even replace those particular activities with new experiences that can be even better.

Adaptation is the key. Mature adults need to adapt in many areas of life, and sexuality is no different. Just as you may now need reading glasses to enjoy reading a good book, so, too, can you enjoy great sex with some simple modifications. Creativity will keep you sexually adventurous through the years. For example, if you love rear-entry penetration but have bad knees, don't worry! There are variations on virtually every sexual position you can imagine, as long as you're open-minded enough to try them. The goal is to allow you to have all the fun you want, but without the pain or other physical limitations that you may be currently experiencing.

BEST POSITIONS FOR BAD KNEES OR HIPS

If you have bad knees or hips, try these variations on some old favorites.

Rear Entry with a Twist

Almost everyone's familiar with the rear-entry or "doggy-style" position, in which the woman is on all fours, and the man enters from behind while on his knees. However, traditional doggy style can be very hard on the woman's knees and wrists, which support the brunt of her weight. For those with arthritis, it can be quite painful, in fact, and many women avoid it for that reason.

To modify the position, the woman stands and places her hands against a wall, bending at approximately a 115-degree angle so that she is standing about 3 feet (1 m) from the wall, hands at shoulder level, with her back straight and legs spread for balance. (She can also lean over a tall counter or a piece of furniture.) Her partner, also standing, can then enter her from behind easily and painlessly. Depending on the height of her partner, she will adjust how far over she bends. She can also bend her knees as far as she is comfortable.

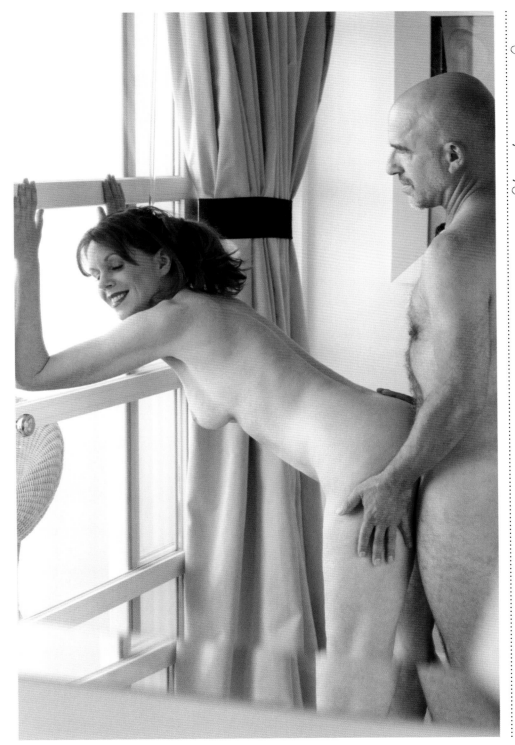

By leaning at an angle, the woman positions her vagina at the right height for penetration; the wall and floor support her weight (with the floor doing most of the work) while her partner thrusts. In fact, she can even just place one hand against the wall and use the other hand to stimulate her clitoris while she's being penetrated, or caress her partner's testicles. Rear-entry penetration also allows for better stimulation of the area commonly known as the G-spot.

Spooning Position

We're all familiar with the concept of spooning, so-called because of its similarity to two spoons resting against each other in a drawer. Taking it the extra step—in which the man lies on his side facing his partner's back, and enters her from behind, can be loads of fun.

If the woman has pain in her hips, she can place a pillow between her knees for support. She can also bend her top leg upward—it still rests on the pillow, with her bottom leg on the bed—to allow him to enter her more easily and take the pressure off her spine.

BEST POSITIONS FOR BAD BACKS

For people experiencing chronic back pain, almost any sexual activity is scary, because even slight movement can induce a high level of pain. Constant pain can dull sexual responses, including delaying and lessening the intensity of orgasm. It can also significantly limit the number of comfortable sexual positions.

Planning is the key. Try practicing yoga or stretching exercises, and take anti-inflammatory medication before sex. You may have to discard traditional positions such as missionary in favor of those that take the pressure off your back and let the mattress support your weight. The partner without the bad back takes the lead and does the majority of the movement.

Face to Face, on a Chair

This position is ideal for women who have back problems, arthritis, or limited mobility. The woman sits on a chair, with a pillow or rolled-up towel between her lower back and the back of the chair. Her partner kneels on the floor, with a pillow under his knees to cushion them; he adds pillows until his penis is at the same level as her vagina. To put less pressure on her back and allow him to enter her more easily, the man holds the woman's knees up to the height of her navel. During sex, he does all of the thrusting. This is an excellent position not only to ease pain but also because it's very intimate, allowing you to gaze into each other's eyes.

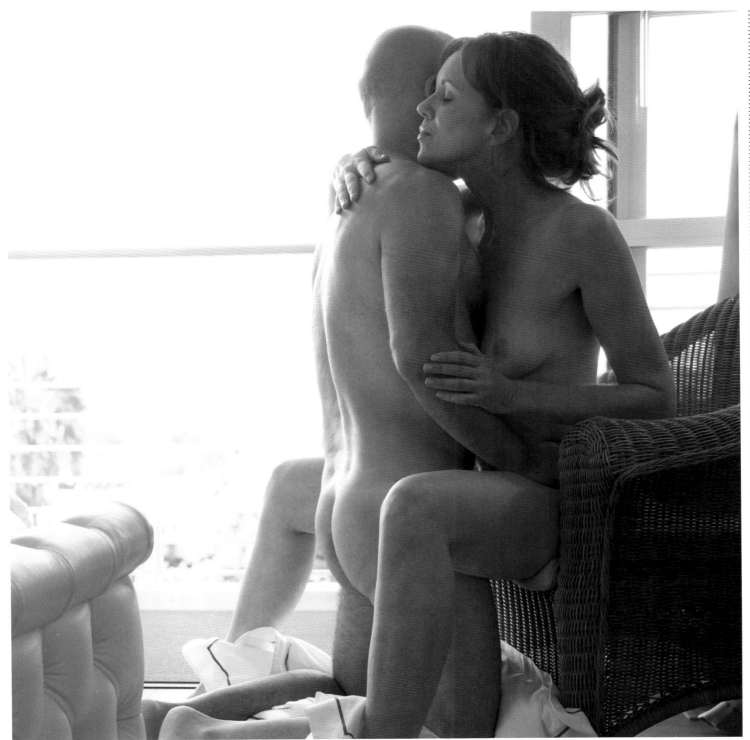

Easy Kama Sutra after Fifty

Reverse Missionary: Female on Top

In this position, the woman sits on her partner, facing away from him, while he's lying flat or sitting in a chair. If he's lying prone, she kneels and lowers herself onto his erection, using her hand to guide him if necessary. During sex, she can adjust herself by leaning forward so that she's almost lying on top of him. This allows her to get more pressure on her clitoris by grinding into his pelvis or using her hand. Her partner can easily stimulate her clitoris if she is in a sitting position.

The woman-on-top position helps the man last longer because he doesn't need to contract his pelvic muscles as much. It's particularly helpful for a woman who has back problems because she doesn't have to support her partner's weight. It's also good for him if he has back issues as his back remains straight and supported. However, this might not be a good position if the woman's knees hurt or she has difficulty keeping her knees bent for a prolonged period. Try placing cushions under your knees to relieve some of the pressure.

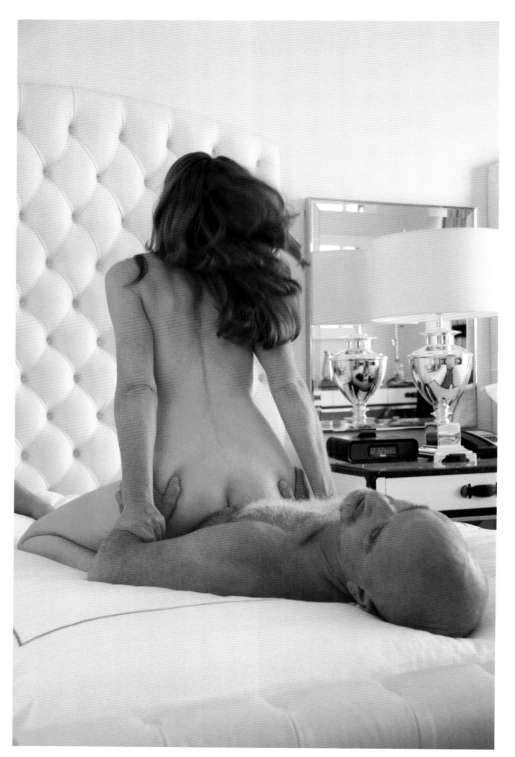

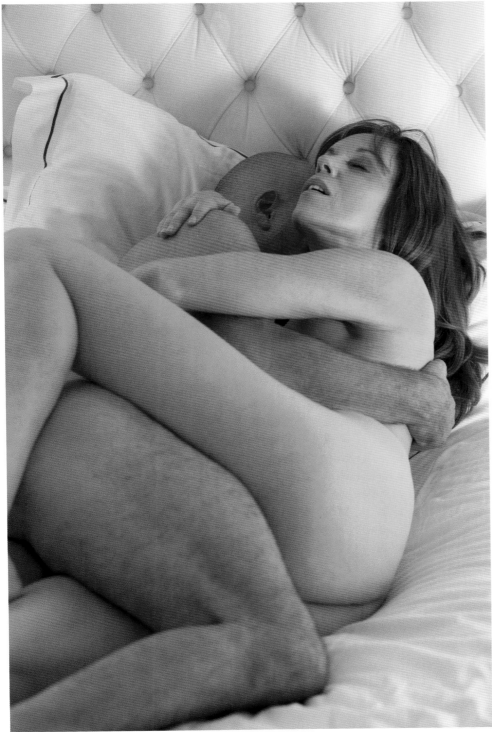

Side to Side, Facing Each Other
With this modification, the couple lies on the bed facing each other as if they were having a conversation. They intertwine their legs so that the woman's top leg (the one not touching the bed) is over the man's top leg. If either one has back problems, he or she can relax and enjoy the ride as the other partner moves his or her hips more. Another benefit of this position is that it promotes increased intimacy—call it cuddling with a twist!

THE BEST POSITION FOR BAD ANYTHING

Non-penetrative sex is the way to go if you want to avoid any kind of strenuous activity. It's also a great option if penetration is not possible because of painful intercourse or erectile dysfunction.

Sixty-Nine

For non-penetrative sex, there exists no more relaxing position than sixty-nine. This oral sex position provides mutual satisfaction because both partners are giving and receiving at the same time! Imagine the shape that the number 69 makes: his face close to her genitals and her face close to his. It can be an appetizer or the main meal.

The different variations of this position allow almost anyone with a physical sensitivity to assume the position that suits him or her best. You can lie prone on the bed while your partner is on top of you (or vice versa), or side to side, which offers support to aching backs or other troublesome bones. You can place pillows, towels, or foam wedges under the body parts that need support, or to offer easier access to your partner's genitals without having to stretch your neck.

For more non-penetrative techniques, turn to chapter 8.

POSITION PROPS YOU CAN USE

Any time you're experiencing pain while having sex, it means that there's pressure being applied to an already problematic area. But just because you're experiencing pain in a certain position doesn't mean you should give up that position. You may find that by tweaking your surroundings a little, you'll enjoy it just as much, or possibly even more, than you did before the pain. Pressure and pain can be greatly alleviated by using a variety of props. You'll need to experiment to discover what works best for you.

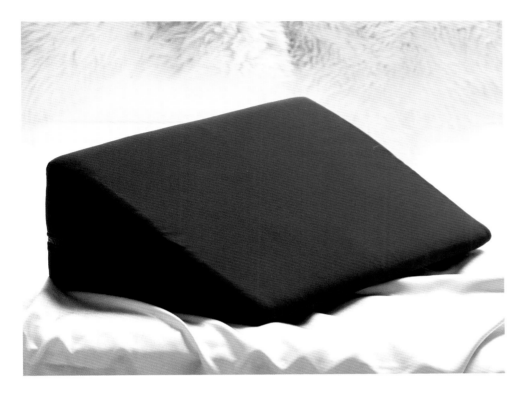

Liberator Wedge

Chairs, Wedges, and Pillows

Believe it or not, even when you're lying flat on your back, you're exerting approximately 55 pounds (25 kg) of pressure on your spine. When you have someone lying on top and thrusting into you with his weight, that 55 pounds (25 kg) could start to feel like 55 tons. Putting pillows or rolled-up towels under your knees cuts the pressure in half! You may also get relief by putting a pillow under your head or your lower back. (By the way, if you're experiencing back pain, you should let your partner do most of the moving.) There is a company (Liberator) that makes foam wedges in all sizes and shapes and also "sex furniture" just for this purpose.

Sex Swing

The sex swing has become a very popular sexual aid over the past few years. Imagine being suspended in a seated position with no body weight to support!

Much like the alternate doggy-style position, the sex swing alleviates pressure on whichever body part would normally be touching the bed, and supports 100 percent of the woman's weight, leaving her free to completely immerse herself in the moment. This Zen-like experience will allow you to "float," while completely focusing and concentrating on the pleasure.

EASY KAMA SUTRA CHECKLIST

Plan your sexual activity.

Take anti-inflammatory medication prior to getting physical.

Take a warm bath.

Do some stretching beforehand.

Decide on a position to try.

Prepare your props (chair, swing, pillows, towels, or foam wedges) so they're close by.

Have lubricant on hand.

If you're not handy, the hardest part about a sex swing will be getting someone to install it! It needs to be affixed to a solid beam that can support your weight and allow for overenthusiastic moments. When hanging your swing, position it so that when the woman is sitting in it, her vagina is at exactly the same height as her partner's penis when he's standing up straight. If it's too high or too low, he'll have to bend his knees or stand on his toes, which completely negates the swing's benefits.

The angle of penetration depends on how far back the woman sits. If she sits farther forward, his penis angles slightly upward and provides more G-spot stimulation, while a downward angle will let his pelvis rub against her clitoris and provide more friction to his penis (which he may need to help him keep his erection harder and longer). You'll have to experiment as a couple because no two people are made exactly the same. Experiment, experiment, experiment!

Just a note of caution: If you suffer from lower back pain, a swing may not be the best option, because the straps usually go around your upper back and below your buttocks. However, you can experiment, because there are many variations in how you can position yourself.

SPECIFIC HEALTH CONCERNS

All of the variations covered so far are the most recommended positions for physical issues that can make intercourse uncomfortable. But certain common illnesses affect sexuality and sexual ability.

After diagnosing an illness, doctors often neglect to give patients information about how their sexuality may be affected, and they sometimes prescribe medications without telling patients about the sexual side effects. This often leads to confusion and frustration. Knowledge truly is power: Armed with proper information, you can greatly decrease the psychological impact of sexual difficulties you may experience as the result of a specific condition.

Diabetes in Men

In men, diabetes can cause difficulty in achieving or maintaining an erection. The disease may cause damage to the erectile tissue, either because of cardiovascular complications that involve clogging of the arteries and, thus, reduce blood flow to the penis, or because of damage to the nerves necessary for erection. You can often overcome this issue by treating the diabetes and with the use of erectile dysfunction medication.

Solution: Please discuss medication and other options with your doctor. You don't need to become celibate just because you have difficulty with erections. That said, did you know that a man *can* have an orgasm even if he doesn't have an erection? His penis can still receive enough stimulation to climax through masturbation or oral sex. So penetration is not the only road to orgasm. Furthermore, as I have said before, sexual satisfaction is not dependent on orgasm, and certainly not on your erection. Remember, you can pleasure her with all your other body parts.

Diabetes in Women

In women, diabetes can cause vaginal dryness as well as loss of sensation. As in men, the lack of blood flow to the genitals as well as nerve damage to the erectile tissues of the clitoris causes these symptoms. The common course of action would be estrogen therapy after a discussion with your doctor. However, there's a simpler fix.

Solution: Lubricants. If you're experiencing dryness without a significant loss of sensation, any good personal lubricant can work wonders. Women are often surprised when they learn that they can solve their problem after spending just a few dollars at the drugstore!

If you *are* experiencing a loss of sensation because of diabetes-related nerve damage, however, look for solutions that increase blood flow to the genitals. Some popular treatment options are:
• Testosterone cream applied to the genitals.
• Sildenafil (Viagra), which can help relax the clitoral and vaginal smooth muscles and increase blood flow.
• An "Eros therapy," a small, FDA-approved pump for the clitoris and external genitalia. It acts much like a penile vacuum pump by drawing blood into the area. Women have reported improved clitoral and genital sensitivity, lubrication, and ability to orgasm with the use of this device.
• A strong vibrating device, such as the Hitachi Magic Wand.

What's of cardinal importance here is that you don't need to suffer in silence. Talk to your doctor and explore your options. Talk to your partner—he'll most certainly be more understanding than you imagine.

CASE STUDY: JONATHAN AND DALIA

Jonathan, fifty-seven, had had a heart attack two years prior to coming to see me at the insistence of his wife. Since his heart attack, he had not only completely avoided sex but all forms of physical contact. He explained that he didn't want to give his wife the idea that he wanted "more" if he caressed or kissed her! He was literally afraid that he would die if he had sex. His wife, Dalia, fifty-two, felt deprived and was growing more and more frustrated.

Interestingly, he had never asked his physician about how and when to resume sexual activity. After reassuring him with some facts (such as the chances of people dying during sex, evidence that sex is good for overall health and for relationships, and that sex could actually prolong his life), I told him to ease back into sexual activity. He started with his wife pleasuring him with her hand and orally, while he did the same for her. With no expectation of intercourse, they were able to move forward. Eventually, they were able to have intercourse without fear or anxiety.

Stroke

A stroke can often impair your ability to move freely, which limits how you have sex and in which positions. Your healthy partner will have to take the reins. Another issue to contend with is the sexual side effects of the medications you may be prescribed to lower your risk of another stroke. Unfortunately, blood pressure medications as well as those prescribed to lower your cholesterol may cause erectile problems.

Solution: Talk to your doctor about ED medications and then explore all the possible props you can use. Try chairs, pillows, a sex swing, foam wedges, and different positions. The severity of the stroke and which body parts are affected will determine which positions you can do. If, for example, one side of your body is partially or fully paralyzed, you may want to position yourself on that side (in order to leave your stronger side free to move and be active) and have your partner be the one doing most of the moving. Try the spooning position, or lie face to face.

Remember that it will take some time, effort, trial and error, and persistence to regain your sexual abilities, just like it has for every other aspect of your rehabilitation.

Heart Attack

If there are any sexual issues following a heart attack, they usually have more to do with a psychological issue than an actual physical one. The culprit? Fear. The thought that the next thrust may be the last can bring on erectile dysfunction in men or vaginal dryness in women. Unfortunately, some men have to take medications following a heart attack to avoid another one (most of the same medications as in stroke), and the side effects of these medications can also be the culprit of sexual problems.

Solution: For the fear: The rule of thumb is that if you're healthy enough to climb a few flights of stairs, you're healthy enough to have sex. And because sex is a cardiovascular activity, it's good for you! Of course, please consult with your doctor following a heart attack to get the "all clear" to have sex. If it makes you feel more mentally at ease, you can ask your partner to do most of the moving, and you can take a more passive (though not less enjoyable!) role. As for the sexual side effects of the medications, please discuss your medical options to treat the erectile dysfunction with your physician.

Arthritis

Even people who have no health concerns sometimes need motivation to get sexual. When you're in pain from arthritis, however, you may have the desire to have sex, but the thought of increasing the pain will more often than not put an end to activity before it starts. The pain may make certain or even all positions uncomfortable or excruciating. Furthermore, many of the medications prescribed to alleviate symptoms may cause sexual side effects such as loss of libido, vaginal dryness, and erectile dysfunction.

Solution: People think they would love to have a spontaneous sex life, but that's not always realistic, nor is it the "be-all and end-all" of sexuality. In fact, some of the best sex you'll ever have is planned (see chapter 6).

CASE STUDY: JAMES AND KATIE

James, sixty-two, has suffered from arthritis for years. Recently, the pain and lack of mobility in his hands has increased, forcing him to change the way he pleasures his wife, Katie, sixty. Because using his hands is more difficult, he now enlists the help of a vibrator to pleasure his wife during foreplay. He also no longer practices the missionary position, as placing pressure on his hands hurts. This couple's preferred position is for him to stand while his wife lies on the edge of the bed with her knees bent. She practices yoga, so she has a lot of flexibility in her hips and legs!

If you have arthritis and suspect you might have sex, why not take anti-inflammatory medication or even a hot bath, hours beforehand? You can also experiment with positions that work for you and use supports that lessen the pressure on the problematic parts of your body. Don't forget your lubricants and, for the man, an ED medication if he wants to engage in penetration.

Most importantly, discuss your concerns with your partner. The more information you share, the higher the level of intimacy. You may want to try positions such as spooning, facing side by side, rear entry with a twist, reverse missionary, or face to face on a chair, all of which allow freedom of movement in a subtle way. Opt for the position that puts the least amount of pressure on the affected area of your body. Remember that you always have the option to engage in non-penetrative sex, as well.

Cancer

Certain cancers are more common with age, such as prostate cancer or breast and other reproductive organ cancers. Sexual problems are common in individuals who are being treated for such cancers. Factors that influence sexual functioning are both psychological and physical in nature. They may include fatigue and other side effects from cancer treatments, anxiety around death, and body image issues. The most common sexual problems for people who have cancer are loss of libido, pain with intercourse, and erectile dysfunction in men. Men may also experience problems with ejaculation. As with diabetes, women may experience loss of genital sensation or difficulty achieving orgasm. Further, medications, such as those used to treat breast cancer, can cause vaginal dryness because they reduce estrogen, which is needed to keep the vaginal walls healthy.

Solution: Sex does not have to involve penile-vaginal intercourse. Especially while going through treatment, you may want to focus less on activities that involve the genitals and more on all-over body caressing and touch. (See chapter 8 for alternatives to intercourse.) This will keep you feeling close and connected, something that will certainly help with your recovery.

A FEW WORDS ON PROSTATE CANCER

For men, the prostate should be routinely checked by a doctor. According to the American Cancer Society, prostate cancer is the most common cancer in American men, with 1 in 6 diagnosed during his lifetime. The average age at the time of diagnosis is about sixty-seven. Prostate cancer is quite rare in men under forty. Fortunately, most men who are diagnosed do not die from it. From a sexual standpoint, men who are treated for prostate cancer will likely experience sexual side effects such as erectile dysfunction and "dry orgasm" (an orgasm without the ejaculation). For some men, erectile functioning may return. It's a good idea to speak to a urologist to discuss how your specific treatment will affect your sexuality.

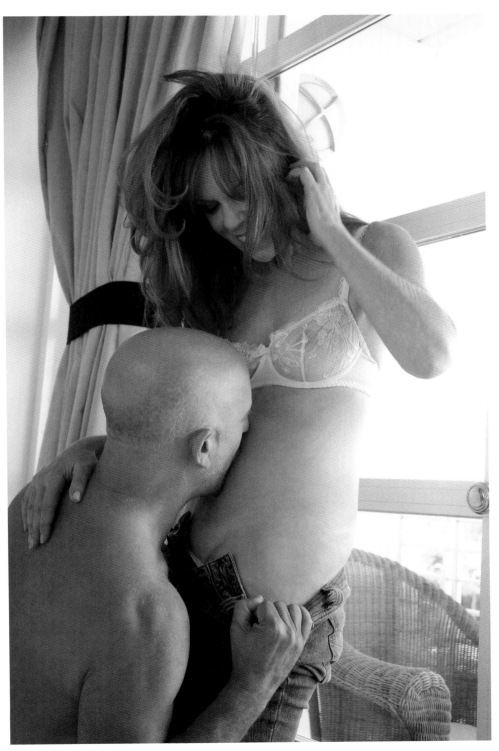

NEW MIND-SETS FOR BETTER SEX

Simply put, when it comes to sex, the only rules are the ones that you set for yourself. Because every person's body is different, so are his or her preferences, dislikes, hang-ups, and fantasies.

You might have had several, or many, sexual partners during the course of your life. They didn't all like or dislike the same things in the bedroom. So what did you do? You adapted. If one move didn't work, you switched it up and tried something different until you found a common ground that pleased you both.

The same applies to sex if you have a physical hurdle to overcome. If doggy style was your thing but now you have bad knees, then rear entry in another position can still do the trick. You have to experiment to know what works with you and your partner in your new reality. Nothing is too silly, and nothing is too "way out there" if it works, satisfies you, and reduces or eliminates your pain. Don't be afraid to write your own new version of the *Kama Sutra*, using only techniques that are compatible with your physical situation.

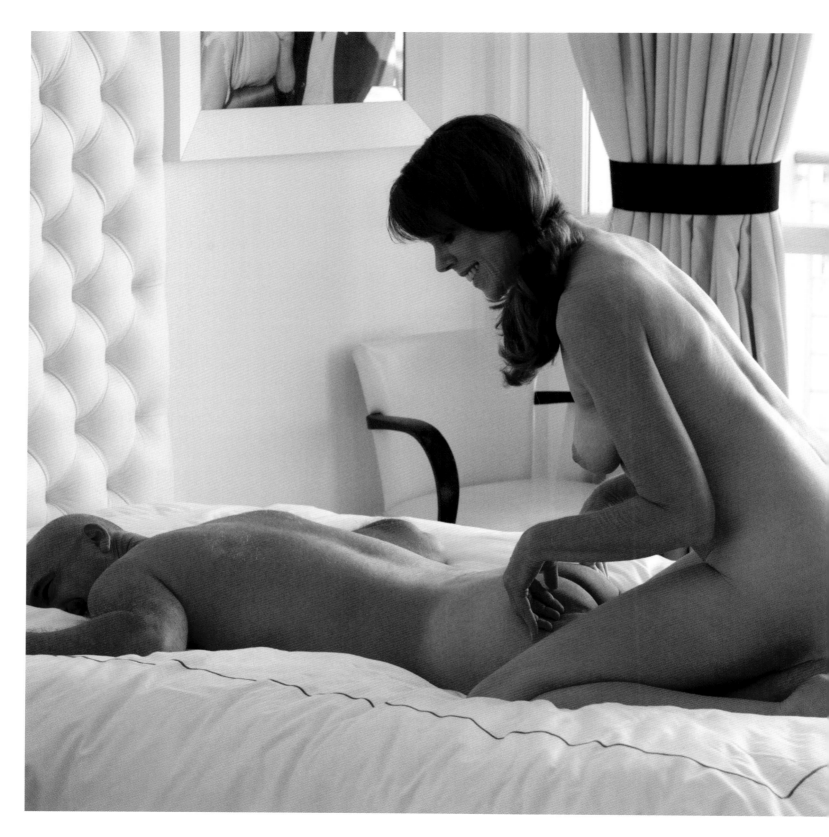

♂08 *Alternatives to Intercourse*

Sex is so much more than just a penis in a vagina! What if your penis isn't hard enough for penetration? What if intercourse is painful because of small tears in your vagina caused by dryness? Do you just give up on sex? NO.

In this chapter, you'll learn how much more you can do with your body to continue to experience sexual pleasure as you grow older. Some things will be activities you may already engage in as foreplay, others may be things you used to do in your earlier years, and some will be completely new to you.

Although many of the activities are described as "alternatives" to intercourse, they're great for foreplay as well. As we age, foreplay becomes more important, as it may take us longer to get aroused and climax. Many of the alternatives described in this chapter offer stimulation to the genitals that's more direct, and therefore more arousing.

THE ART OF ORAL SEX

One of the best—and certainly most popular—alternatives to intercourse is oral sex. Though it's great at any age, it has tons of benefits for people over fifty, as well. For example, a mature man may need more constant and direct stimulation of the penis to get and stay hard, in part because blood is flowing more slowly into his penis. That's because as he ages, fatty substances (plaques) form inside the tiny arteries of his penis, which impairs blood flow to the organ. If it takes him a little longer to get a full erection, oral sex is a great way to get him harder. And if done for its own sake, fellatio relieves the pressure on him to get a full erection and to maintain it for penetration, especially if he has ED. Remember, a man can still have an orgasm and ejaculate, even if he doesn't have an erection!

In addition, some postmenopausal women complain of feeling less sensation in their clitoris than they did before menopause, due to the drastic reduction in estrogen production. (Not all women experience this, just as not all women experience hot flashes.) At this point in their sex lives, they may find that they, like their men, need the additional stimulation that oral sex provides.

GOING DOWN ON HER

Men, don't assume that what worked for her twenty years ago still works today. Here's the best way to find out what does: ASK! Ask her questions such as:

• Does she feel anything at all from your tongue?
• What kind of pressure feels best: a light touch or more intense, direct pressure?
• Does she need you to apply pressure with your hand or finger as well?
• Does she like attention to other erogenous zones—such as her inner thighs, labia, or anus?

If she needs more pressure, you can also use your tongue, your lips, and your fingers—or all of them—at the same time to stimulate her fully.

Ready to get creative? Here are some other moves to try that provide added stimulation:

The finger flick-and-lick: While your mouth is on her clitoris, gently insert a lubricated index finger into her vagina. With your palm facing upward, use your finger to make a "come here" motion. This massages the anterior wall of her vagina, otherwise known as the G-spot.

Tongue writing: Instead of licking in circles, pretend that you're using your tongue as a pen and write numbers or the alphabet on her clitoris.

The side-to-side tease: When you get to the area, instead of just "diving in," go back and forth, kissing from thigh to thigh, each time teasing her clitoris with a short puff of hot breath. Each time you pass over it, she'll think you are going to lick it, until the tension and excitement are so high that it won't take her long to reach orgasm.

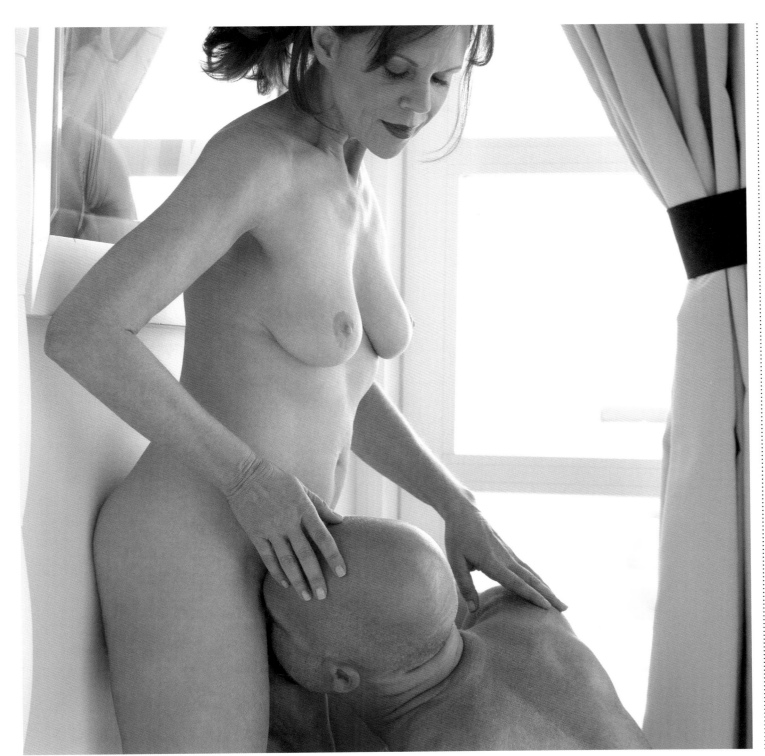

Use a warmed glass dildo: There are many beautiful dildos made of glass available on the market. They can be immersed in warm water for a few minutes to reach the same temperature as a penis. You can keep one in a bowl of warm water next to the bed, and when the time is right, it can be inserted in the vagina, while you are simultaneously licking her clitoris. She will get dual stimulation, and she will love it.

The big tease: Using your finger, pull the hood of her clitoris back, exposing it. Lick all around the clitoris and labia but don't actually make contact with the clitoris. Come very close to it, and every once in a while make gentle, almost indirect contact, until she's pushing your head into it! Anticipation is half the battle and three-fourths the fun.

Don't forget that only your partner can show you the best way to please her. Check in with her every so often to make sure she likes what you're doing. If she's shy about telling you, encourage her to vocalize her pleasure.

Modify Your Positions

To avoid neck strain, have her elevate her pelvic area with pillows or a foam wedge (such as the Liberator) under her buttocks in order to make her genitals more accessible. Her vulva should be at your face level. The best position for this is with you kneeling at her feet while she's seated on the edge of the bed or a chair. To alleviate knee strain, place pillows under your own knees. If bending your knees is not ideal, then you can lie down with your head toward her feet, and your face aligned with her vulva—as if you were doing 69.

Another option is to have her lie on her back with her legs straight and apart, or with her knees slightly bent if this causes no discomfort, and you on your stomach between her legs. She may need to prop up her pelvis with pillows so that her vulva and your face are at the same level. This should cause little or no strain to your knees or your neck, but your feet or part of your legs may dangle off the bed.

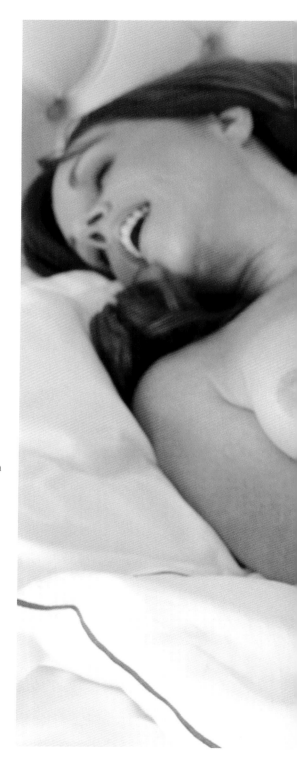

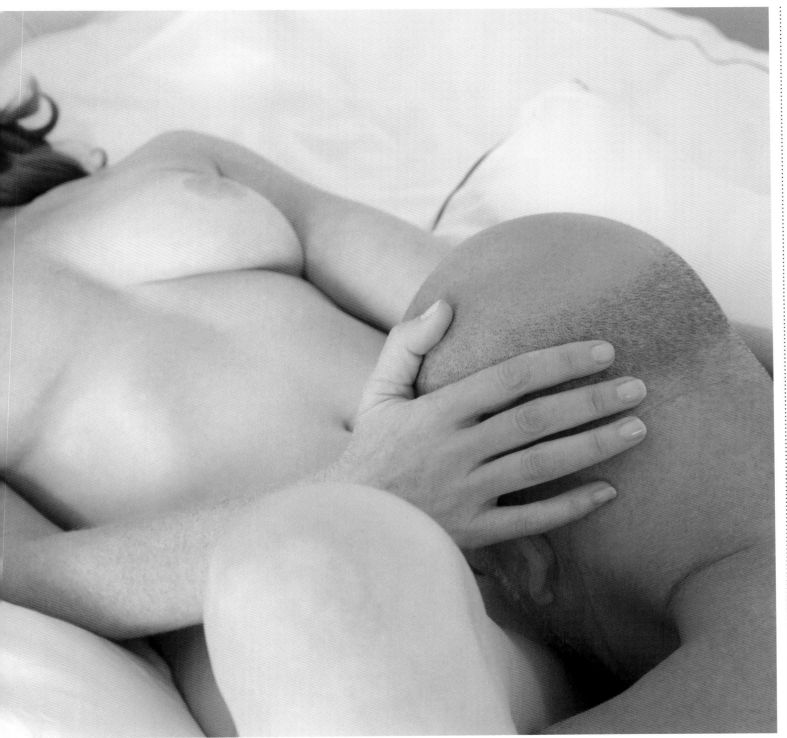

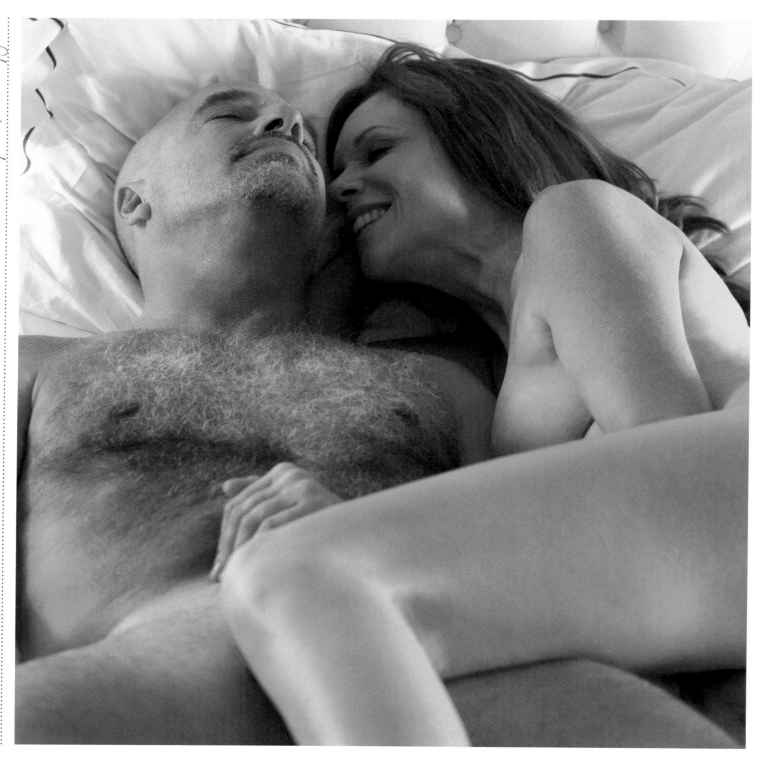

GOING DOWN ON HIM

Mature men can feel a sense of shame if they can't "perform" as they once could—but they shouldn't! I've found that most women completely understand, so ladies, reassure your man that going down on him is simply to give him pleasure rather than preparing him for intercourse. Assure him that an erection doesn't have to be the goal. (He'll enjoy your mouth on his penis no matter what!) And men, do your part by assuring her that your lack of erection isn't related to your attraction to her or her technique.

A Flaccid Penis Can Still Be Fun

In his younger years, just the thought of a blow job may have been enough to give your partner a solid erection. In his later years, however, it may take a lot more. And he may not be able to get an erection at all because of medical issues. Don't assume he isn't enjoying your efforts if he doesn't get hard.

But that doesn't mean that a flaccid penis is a useless penis. You can still have fun with it, and he'll still get enjoyment out of the experience. The advantage of performing oral sex on a flaccid penis is that it's easy to take the whole thing in your mouth. You also have more flexibility with it while it's there. You can stretch it, roll it around, or squeeze it with your lips.

Getting Him Hard

The fact that it takes him longer to get erect is in no way a sign that you're not arousing him. Be patient, and just have fun. If you try too hard, he may feel pressured to get there, and this will impede his ability to get or maintain an erection. For the majority of men, your mouth on his penis feels great. But simply licking and sucking him may not be enough.

Use your hand: While you're using your tongue and your lips to pleasure him, stroke his shaft with your hand, mimicking the movements he'd make if he were masturbating. To blow his mind, try sucking him with the same rhythm at the same time, as if your hand were an extension of your mouth. Allow your saliva to flow freely from your mouth to lubricate and warm your hand.

Use massage oil: Having his genitals gently massaged with a very slippery oil (Nuru oil is amazing) is both very relaxing in and of itself, and very exciting. This can be done even without the premise of impending sex, but purely for relaxation. More often than not it will excite him.

Shave him: Any man who has ever had his genitals shaved will tell you that aside from feeling great, it's an immense turn-on. When he's soft and smooth down there, every sensation seems to be amplified. Bonus for the woman is that it's cleaner and there are no pubic hairs to spit out.

Do something out of character: Many men will never tell their woman that they like something she never does, out of fear that they will seem perverted or kinky. They say that familiarity breeds contempt, so why not learn a few new tricks? Whether it be sexy lingerie, dirty talk, or a strip tease, make him feel like he's going to bed with a new woman. Doing something that you've never tried will turn him on all on its own.

Don't forget the other "bits": Lavish attention on the head of his penis, frenulum (that little piece of skin on the underside, below the head), and shaft. Lick his testicles or take them in your mouth. Don't forget to show his perineum—the space between his testicles and his anus—some action as well with gentle pressure or soft strokes.

Modify Your Positions

Take his penis in your mouth while you lay your head on his belly—a perfect spot to rest your head if you need a little break. It's also ideal if his penis curves upward. You may find yourself lying perpendicular to his body. In this position, he can be completely relaxed with no pressure on his back, especially if he puts a pillow under his knees. If his penis tends to point downward, climb on top of him, facing his feet, as if you were going to do 69. You can rest on your knees and elbows, rocking back and forth as he slips in and out

of your mouth. Or, try pleasuring him while he's sitting in a chair, with you sitting or kneeling between his feet. Use supporting pillows for your own knees, if necessary.

Swallow, Spit, or Neither?

Most of us can think back to adolescent conversations about sex that invariably included jokes about women swallowing ejaculate. Unfortunately, these comments often led women to believe that all men expect them to swallow. When they were younger, they thought swallowing semen was expected of them.

But as women get older, they're often more inclined to take charge of their sexuality. Many women decide that swallowing isn't something they want to do. They also learn that their partner doesn't care. It's not that it wouldn't feel nice for him to finish while in a warm, wet place—it's just that it's not necessary for him to enjoy the experience.

Before you decide what to do with his ejaculate, consider this fact: As men age, they ejaculate less, and less forcefully. This may influence your decision. Basically, you have three options:
• If you're not comfortable having him ejaculate in your mouth, take his penis out and finish the job with your hand (make sure he tells you when he's about to come).
• If you are comfortable with him ejaculating in your mouth, you can swallow.
• If you want to allow him to ejaculate in your mouth but don't want to swallow, have a tissue nearby so that you can subtly spit it out.

Do what feels good for you.
There are NO RULES.

The Gag Reflex

As we age, some of us develop digestive issues or problems with the respiratory system that can affect the gag reflex, making it more sensitive. Thus, where at one time "deep throating" was possible, it may now take a little more work and adaptation to take in much of the penis.

The best way to adapt is to practice taking in more and more of his penis a little bit at a time. Remember to supplement your mouth and tongue with your hand on his shaft. Practice on a Popsicle or a banana if you want to prepare yourself to surprise him with deeper oral penetration.

During oral sex, breathe through your nose, relax your throat muscles, and only insert his penis as deeply as you can without triggering your gag reflex. If you're gagging, then you've gone too far for now, so ease up a bit. With time, you'll get used to it and will be able to get it deeper. Once there, try "swallowing" with him inside—it will drive him wild.

PLEASURE IN HAND

Most people masturbate regularly, whether they're in a relationship or not, no matter their age. In fact, the groundbreaking Kinsey Reports of 1948 and 1953 found that, respectively, almost 40 percent of men and 30 percent of women in relationships masturbated. Though societal attitudes toward sex have evolved since those studies

were conducted—indeed, over the course of our lifetimes!—more contemporary surveys paint a similar picture. An article titled "Masturbation in the United States" published in the *Journal of Sex and Marital Therapy* reported that 38 percent of women and 61 percent of men (aged eighteen to sixty) masturbated in the past year. Further, the 2009 National Survey of Sexual Health and Behavior, of people between fourteen and ninety-four, found that between 28 and 69 percent of men (depending on age) masturbated in the last month. Let's face it: It's a pleasurable habit that would be hard to give up (and why would you want to?), and it is in fact very healthy because it increases blood flow to the genitals.

I Do Me, You Do You

Masturbating together as a couple can be a tremendous turn-on and is also a wonderful way for each partner to know exactly how the other likes to be touched. The voyeur/exhibitionist theme can be a very powerful aphrodisiac that I've heard described by those who practice masturbating together as even more intimate than actual lovemaking. It has something to do with the feeling of vulnerability when engaging in an act that's usually reserved for when you are alone. Of course, there's nothing that prevents you from adding a helping hand, finger, or tongue. You set your own rules.

The Best Way to Give Him a Hand

Another alternative to penetrative sex is mutual masturbation. It can be a great appetizer or the main course! The sliding of her lubricated hand up and down his shaft while he simultaneously slips a lubricated finger around her vulva and into her vagina can make both partners feel like they are teenagers again. Also, try these sexy tips:

• Use lubricant.
• If he isn't circumcised, pull the skin upward rather than back.
• Start by encircling your fingers (thumb and index) at the base and move up.
• Caress the head of the penis and play with the testicles with your other hand.
• When he's erect, move your hand up and down, going all the way up past the penis head and all the way down to the firm base.
• Ask him whether he likes to be stroked fast or slow, and whether he prefers a firm or lighter hold.

LOVEMAKING FROM BEHIND

According to a 2010 paper published in the *Journal of Sex Research*, more than 40 percent of heterosexual adults have tried anal sex, and up to 10 percent of heterosexual adults have done it at least once in the previous year. Further, a *Redbook* magazine survey of 100,000 women found that 43 percent of married women have tried anal intercourse. So with this many people having at least tried anal sex, we can assume that it's not as taboo a behavior as we have been led to believe.

In fact, I have met many heterosexual couples who practice it regularly. Many weren't able to engage in vaginal intercourse because she experienced severe pain with penetration, but they still derived tremendous pleasure from the experience of anal sex. The men told me that they don't feel "deprived" of intercourse at all when this is an option.

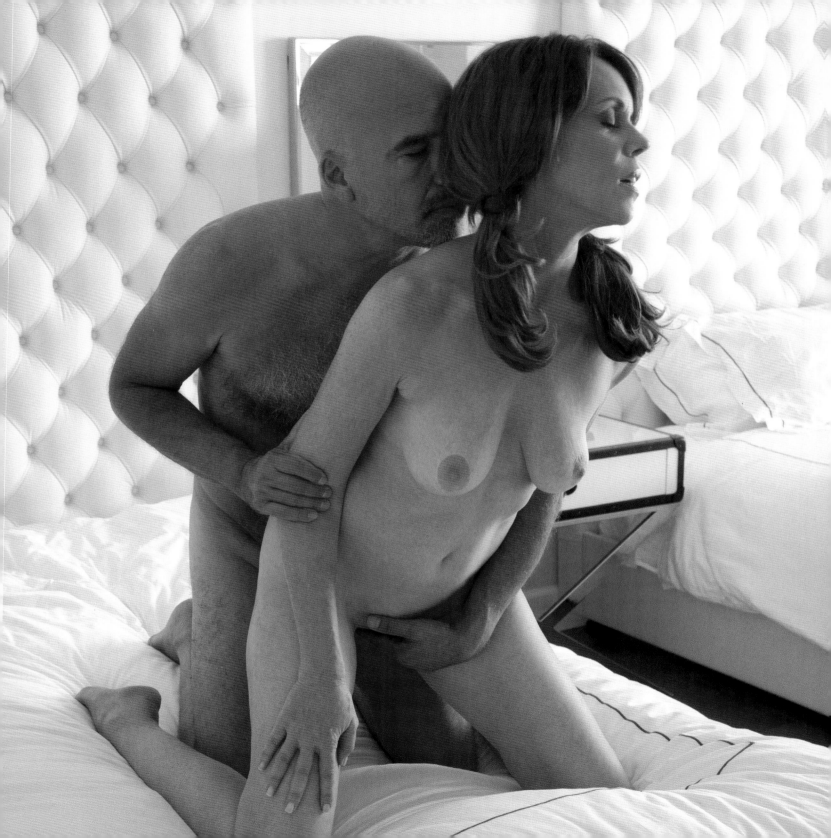

A word of caution: Don't go from anal penetration to vaginal penetration without washing the penis first, because you'll be transferring unwanted bacteria.

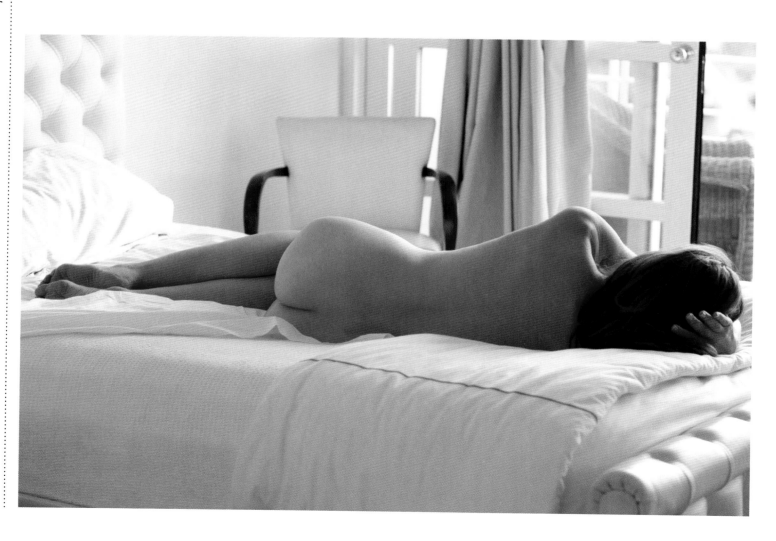

Although it might seem that it's the man who would get the most pleasure from anal sex, women can and do enjoy it, too. According to Jack Morin, Ph.D., author of *Anal Pleasure and Health: A Guide for Men, Women, and Couples*, in both men and women the anus is actively involved during arousal. It, too, when stimulated, gets congested with blood and contracts, as does the vagina. What's more, there are many nerve endings in the anal muscles and the perineum (the area between the genitals and the anus) that are very sensitive to touch. Some women really enjoy rectal massage in combination with G-spot stimulation. Only you can decide whether anal sex is something that appeals to you and your partner.

If you're about to try anal sex for the first time, here are a few tips for success.
• Go very slowly.
• Use ample amounts of lubrication—unlike the vagina, the rectum doesn't produce its own lubrication.
• Start by inserting a lubricated finger.
• Before any sort of penetration, she should "bear down" rather than contract her pelvic floor (like she might do with Kegel exercises).
• Slowly move up to inserting your penis.
• Check in with her frequently. If it's too painful, stop.

Sometimes as we age, we begin to experience digestive difficulties (think hemorrhoids or difficulty with bowel control) that could interfere with feeling pleasure from anal stimulation. If this is your case, anal sex might not be an option for you. If you do choose to engage in anal sex, make sure your partner knows about these issues to help manage unforeseen surprises.

What If He Wants Some Anal Play?

Many men enjoy a little penetrative anal play. If your man is one of them, it *does not* mean he's gay, nor does it imply that he wants a penis inserted in his rectum. Both men and women have many nerve endings in the anal area that can provide sexual pleasure. A finger, vibrator, or dildo inserted into his anus can stimulate his prostate gland. Try circling his anus with your lubricated finger, then inserting it a little bit at a time. The sensations provided by prostate massage can cause mind-blowing orgasms.

Many men and women find oral-anal play (also known as analingus or "rimming") to be pleasurable. Before going into that area, check to make sure your partner feels at ease with it. Thoroughly wash the anal region to remove most external fecal particles and reduce the risk of bacterial infection. Using a barrier such as a dental dam (or cutting a latex condom down the middle) also reduces the risk of infection. Never go from licking the anus to the vagina, as you risk a urinary tract infection or worse.

SEX TOYS AND WOMEN

Seventy-eight percent of women who use sex toys are in a relationship.

Ninety percent of women said they were comfortable talking to their partner about sex toys.

One in five women masturbates at least once a week.

Women who use sex toys report experiencing higher levels of sexual function and satisfaction with their partners than non-users.

Sex toy users also find it easier to reach orgasm when compared with non-users.

Source: The Berman Center, Chicago, 2004.

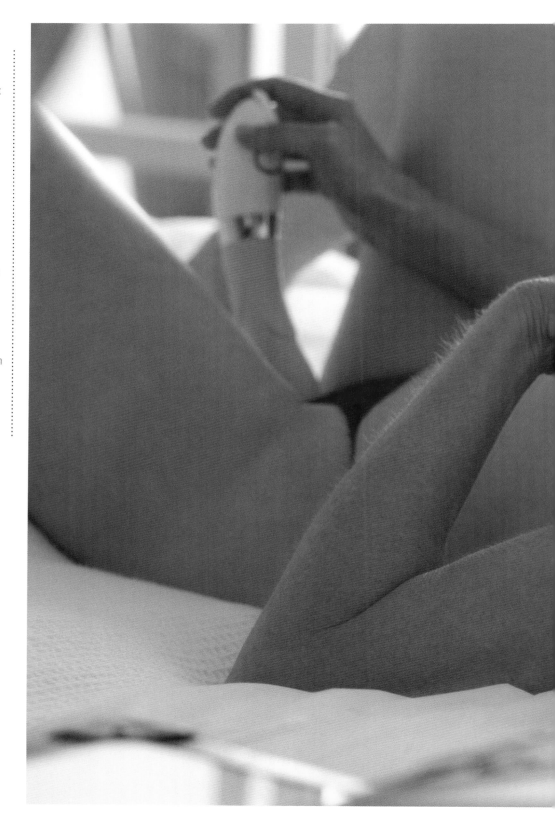

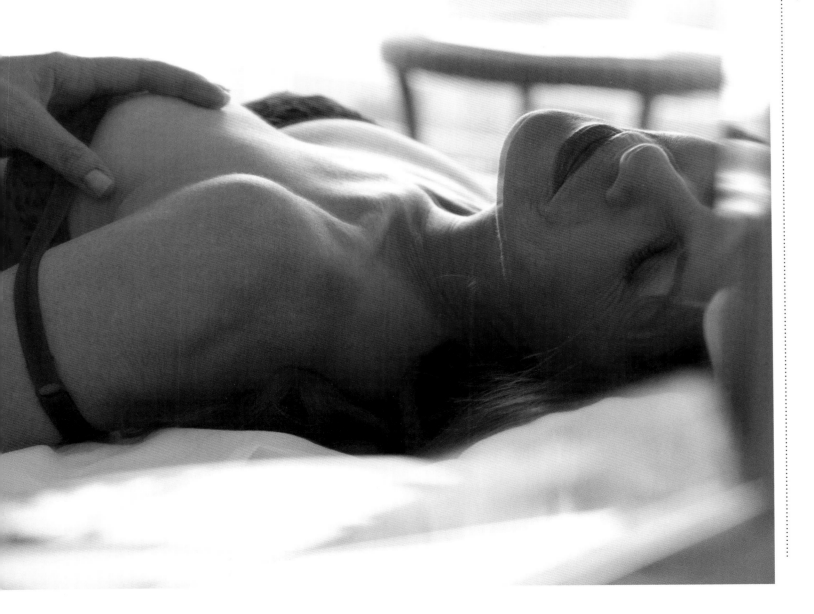

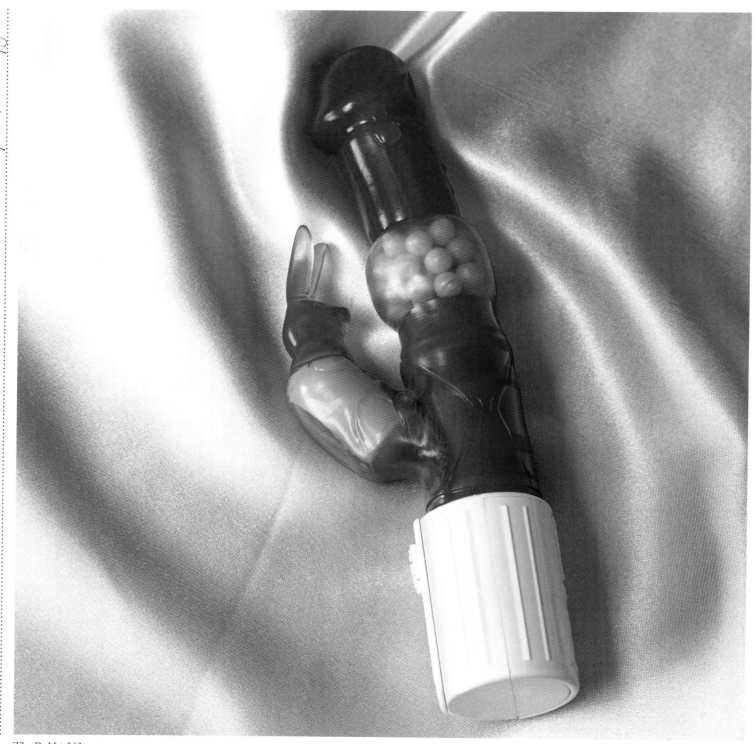

The Rabbit Vibrator

THE INS AND OUTS OF SEX TOYS

In the early twentieth century, doctors used medical devices (really an early form of vibrators) to treat women with "hysteria." It seems the orgasms that resulted calmed the women. More recently, the use of sex toys was seen as a sign of nymphomania in women and inadequacy in men. Thankfully, we see things very differently today! Sex toys can enhance any sex life, and it really doesn't matter whether you're single or in a relationship. There's absolutely no shame whatsoever in using them on a regular or even frequent basis, because the bottom line is they're fun and they feel good!

But keep in mind that toys can't replace human intimacy. If your partner wants to use a sex toy, it doesn't mean that you're replaceable in any way. Partners' desire to use a sex toy has less to do with you, and more to do with their attempt to meet their own needs. And, as in mutual masturbation, think how hot it can be to watch your partner pleasure him- or herself!

Myths and Facts about Sex Toys

Myth: Only single women use sex toys.
Fact: Almost 50 percent of women use sex toys or have tried them in the past, and women in relationships are even more likely to use them.

Myth: Only younger women use sex toys.
Fact: Women aged fifty-five to sixty are just as likely as younger women to have tried a sex toy at some point in their lives.

Myth: If you use a sex toy, it means you're dissatisfied with partner sex.
Fact: Sex-toy users are significantly more likely to report a higher level of desire and interest in sex, and less pain during and following intercourse according to a 2004 Berman Center study.

Batteries, Please . . .

One of the benefits of using a sex toy as we grow older is that it can help do some of the "heavy lifting," so to speak. From a purely practical standpoint, a sex toy can help you achieve results that otherwise might be uncomfortable, unlikely, or impossible. In addition to using a sex toy to bring on climax, a battery-operated helper can get the juices flowing, allowing the partners to finish up "in person." Consider the following:
• If you have trouble maintaining an erection, you can use a vibrator or dildo on her to give her the added stimulation she may want if you cannot "finish the job."
• Use a cock ring with vibrating bullet. This will keep you harder longer and will provide added clitoral stimulation for her.

• If you have arthritis in your hands and fingers, dildos or clitoral stimulators can help you stimulate your partner. You can always jump in at any time and replace the toy with the love machine that is attached to your body! If you can't achieve an erection, a hollow strap-on penis can do the job, allowing you to get the benefit of pleasuring your partner through the penetration that she wants.

Take a trip to the closest sex shop to see what catches your eye. If you're uncomfortable walking into a brick-and-mortar building, go online! There are thousands of websites selling a huge variety of sexual aids, and there's sure to be one for you. My personal favorites are www.goodforher.com, www.goodvibrations.com, www.comeasyouare.com, and www.joytoyz.com.

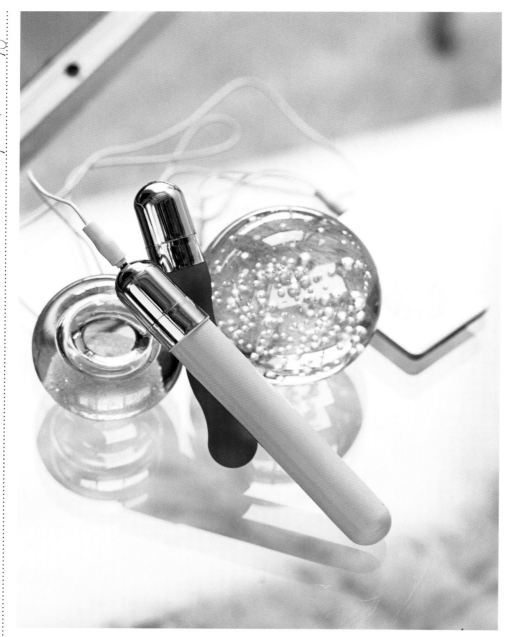

Vibrators come in a variety of shapes, colors, and textures.

Toys for Women

Dildos: A dildo is shaped like an erect penis. This toy is most commonly used for vaginal or anal penetration and can be used with or without a partner. There are many types of dildos that vary in texture, shape, and color.

Vibrators: Vibrators are simply dildos that vibrate (see photos at left and opposite top right). Some vibrators are meant to be used vaginally, others stimulate the clitoris, and some do both. The most common vibrator (popularized by the television show *Sex in the City*) is the Rabbit (see page 130), so-called because it has two little vibrating "ears" that stimulate the clitoris while the shaft of the vibrating dildo rotates inside the vagina.

Clitoral stimulators: These toys come in all shapes, but they are usually no bigger than your palm (they're sometimes referred to as "bullets"). Some are really cute (such as the Hello Kitty Pocket Rocket), are no bigger than a lipstick, and fit nicely into a purse. Others are curved (see photo opposite top left). Most are battery operated, and some even have remote controls!

G-spot stimulators: These are vibrators that are curved so that they can easily reach your G-spot, an area on the anterior wall of the vagina (the side toward the belly button). There are hundreds of models on the market today.

Toys for Men

Penis rings: Also known as "cock rings," these are placed around the base of the penis once it's erect. This is a great toy for men who have trouble maintaining an erection. Penis rings squeeze the penis (comfortably), essentially trapping blood in it, which allows for a longer-lasting erection.

Artificial penis "sleeves": These are—just like they sound—sleeves made of rubber or silicone into which a man inserts his penis and thrusts or squeezes (see bottom photo at right).

Toys for Both

Men can also use vibrators to massage the perineum. Both men and women can use butt plugs for anal stimulation. And some toys can be used simultaneously by both men and women—such as penis rings that have a vibrating "bullet" attached that stimulates a woman's clitoris at the same time or the We-Vibe, which can be used during intercourse. It stimulates her G-spot and clitoris while providing sensations for him, too.

Go Green!

Demand is hot for green sex toys. With the growing popularity of the green lifestyle, more and more companies are offering environmentally friendly options for sex. If you're a woman over fifty, it's also a great idea to use the least amount of chemicals in your vagina as possible, because it may be more sensitive, just like the skin on your face. Some examples of "eco-rotica" include:

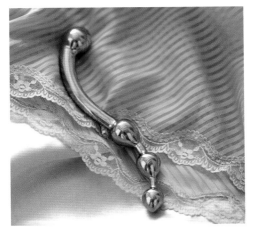

Clitoral Stimulator

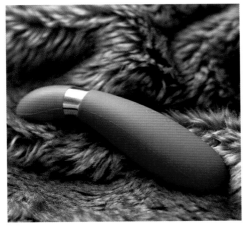

Vibrator

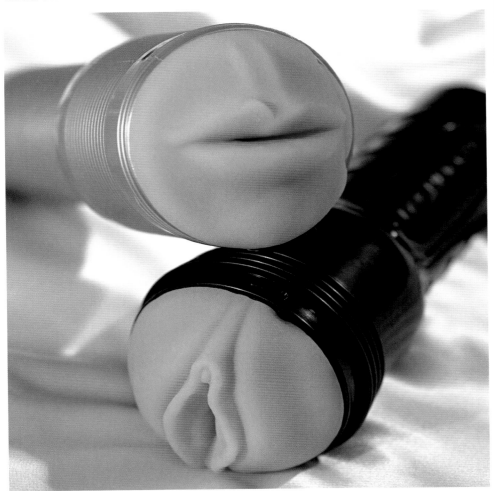

Penis Sleeves

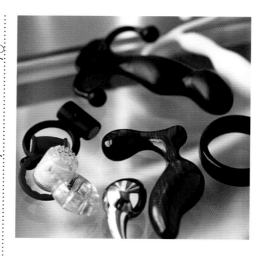

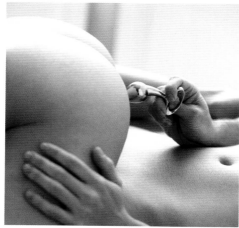

*Sex toys can enhance any relationship—
they're fun and they feel good!*

Lubricants:
• Aloe Cadabra Natural Aloe Unscented
Lubricant: Organic plant-based lubricant
(www.aloecadabra.com)
• Yes Natural Lubricants: Water- and
oil-based lubricants that are chemical and
preservative free (www.yesyesyes.org)
• Good Clean Love: Organic lubricants,
body candies, and love oil (www.
goodcleanlove.com)

Condoms:
• Glyde Condoms: Plant-based, vegan-
friendly condoms made from natural rubber
that are free from animal by-products and
animal testing (www.glydeamerica.com)

Sex Toys:
• Earth Erotics: Vegan sex toys such as
vibrators, anal toys, dildos, and lubricants
(www.eartherotics.com/catalog)
• The Vegan Sex Shop: A website that lists
many of the available vegan sex toys such as
butt plugs, vibrators, lingerie, candles, and
more (www.thevegansexshop.com)

THE POWER OF TOUCH: SENSUAL MASSAGE

Although some couples practice massage
on a regular basis, most people have to
think back to the initial dating stage of their
relationship to remember the last time they
massaged their partner. The older we get,
the likelier we are to experience aches and
pains. A gentle massage can go a long way
to alleviate these. As a bonus, a massage will
make you feel close to your partner, while
arousing him or her at the same time!

Low lighting, candles, soft music, and
incense can all help set the mood. Buy
some good massage oil, and if you're so
inclined, you can actually pick up a pretty
good folding massage table for about $200.
A massage table makes it much easier to
massage someone at the right height. You can
walk around the table to get to all the right
places. The added advantage to a massage
table is that it's also the perfect height for sex!

Want a Happy Ending with That?
Don't necessarily think of a massage as a
means to an end (sex), but rather enjoy it
for what it is: sensual touching. Perform a
complete full-body massage on your partner:
Attend to every part of his or her body—
fingers, toes, neck, arms, etc.—leaving the
genitals until the end.

A massage can be as simple as light touching.
Use your fingertips and fingernails to very
lightly and barely touch the skin, sending
shivers and a tickling sensation across your
partner's skin. Or your sensual massage can
be more intense. Let your partner decide
what works for him or her. Ask your partner
to guide you by letting you know what kind
of touching he or she likes. Once you've
attended to the whole body, you can get to
the genitals and stimulate your partner to a
"happy ending" (orgasm) or two!

> If you want the candle in your relationship to always be lit, make it a point to never go to sleep before kissing your partner soulfully. It makes waking up in the morning next to him or her all that much better.

Keep in mind a few considerations. You or your partner may have joint pain, or certain areas of the body that are very sensitive to any kind of pressure. Always start off slowly and gently, and frequently check in with your partner to make sure you are touching in the way that's most comfortable.

CUDDLING AND KISSING

The longer we're with someone in a relationship, the more we tend to settle into a comfort zone, and the more we overlook some of the details that actually got us into the relationship in the first place. That's why cuddling and kissing are so important!

Mature men tend to be more eager to explore nonsexual touching than they were in their younger years, and such activity can at times be enough for them. Kissing, whether you like it slow and delicate or deep with nibbles and bites, can be such a turn-on. It almost always leads to more—but it doesn't have to. The same goes for cuddling, which you can do clothed or naked, complete with slow, deliberate caresses to the erogenous zones.

When embracing your partner for a cuddle, pay attention to any physical condition that may cause him or her discomfort and that may require a more tender caress.

YES, IT DOES COUNT AS SEX

Keep in mind that as we age, we require an increasing amount of stimulation to get our juices flowing. This is because of a combination of the physical aging process and the reality that mentally, after what could potentially be thousands of sexual experiences over the span of our lifetimes, we've often done the same things over and over. With this in mind, it's entirely normal to want to vary your sexual menu, just as you would your dinner menu. And regardless of what it is that pleases your palate, rest assured—it's all nourishing!

10 SENSUAL MASSAGE TIPS AND TRICKS

Do the massage on a blanket or towel that you don't mind getting stained with oil.

The more oil or lotion you use, the better. You can go natural with olive or coconut oil or use store-bought massage oil.

Start with your partner lying on his or her stomach. Save the front for last.

Don't go deep at first. Keep your touch light, focusing on long strokes rather than deep-tissue rubbing, so that you can last longer than 5 minutes.

You take control of the body. Your partner doesn't move at all.

Don't stay just on one part of the body. Move around.

Resist participating. Just think of pleasing your partner. It's all about him or her.

Listen to your partner's breath. When it increases, increase your pace, or slow it down if you want it to last longer.

Stand at your partner's feet and glide up both legs to the genitals.

Tease, tease, tease. Get close to the genitals or touch them lightly, then move to another body part and repeat.

Remember, the journey is the pleasure.

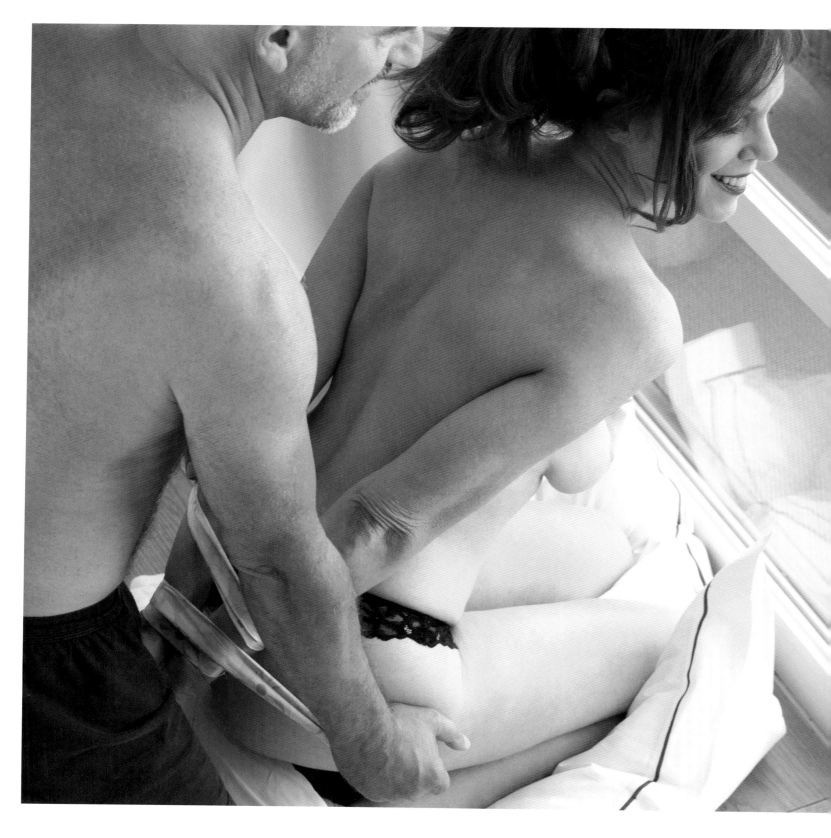

09 *Stretching Your Boundaries*

After people spend years together as a couple, it's easy to see how boredom can set in. Sex can be good, even satisfying, but the "spice" is gone. So couples often look for tips and ideas about how they can have better and more exciting sex. If we relied on media portrayals, we'd associate adventurous sex with youth, but that's not always the case. Oftentimes, couples in their middle years and beyond are very open to pushing sexual boundaries, whether it involves role-play, bondage, props, or including a third party. Being comfortable with themselves and their partners provides a foundation to explore new activities in their sex lives.

FANTASY AND ROLE-PLAYING

The longer we're together, the greater the chance of sexual boredom setting in. That's because the longer we're together, the more we know our partner, and when we know our partner inside out, the mystery is gone. But mystery is what breeds passion. So when we role-play, we take on a different persona—one that's new to our partner.

In a fantasy, you can be whomever you want, act however you want, and have your partner behave in any way you want. Role-playing lets you bring your fantasies to life. You're the director of your own erotic play!

Role-playing is about more than just sex, however. It keeps the fire burning, yes, but it also requires you to communicate, trust each other, care about each other's needs, and work together as a team. These are all great qualities that help make relationships work and increase the level of intimacy.

Please bear in mind that fantasies are just that—fantasies. If you fantasize about your partner seducing you or "forcing" sex on you, it doesn't mean that you actually want to be raped. Nor are fantasies threats to the relationship. If your partner's fantasy involves you pretending to be a stripper, it doesn't imply he wants to leave you for one. Please reassure each other that this is merely a fantasy, and that you want your partner, and your partner alone. As you can see, communication is key for successful role-playing and fantasy sharing.

Here's something to consider if you have a long history together: Be mindful of any past hurts that role-playing or sharing fantasies may trigger. For example, if as a couple you've dealt with cheating behavior in the past (and have since healed from it), you wouldn't want to role-play a fantasy that involved infidelity.

Your Role-Playing Bag of Tricks

• Go online for great ideas (try www.thefantasybox.com), watch porn with storylines, or read erotic novels.

• Come up with your roles or characters: teacher/student, nurse/patient, superhero/damsel in distress, subordinate/master, or stripper/client—whatever sounds the most fun to you!

• Decide on a scenario: bar pickup/seduction, in a doctor's office, etc.

• Give your partner some instruction as to how you'd like him or her to act in the scene.

• Get into costume and into character. Shopping for your costumes together can create some juicy anticipation—or you can have tons of fun surprising each other!

• Have fun and make sure you're both comfortable—know your boundaries.

• You can act out your fantasy over the course of an evening or a whole day.

• Establish a "safe" word to stop your role-playing if you're no longer feeling comfortable.

GETTING KINKY WITH BDSM

BDSM stands for bondage, dominance/ discipline, sadism/submission, and masochism. It's is a form of consensual sexual play that involves giving and receiving various sensations. As the term implies, *bondage* refers to playing with restraints. Dominance/discipline, sadism/submission, and masochism refer to one person submitting while the other dominates. Many people experience a thrill when they let go of all control in a sexual situation and completely submit to their partner.

Incorporating a little BDSM into your sexual repertoire can increase your levels of arousal. If you've never ventured into this area, now is as good a time as any. If you've played with BDSM before, bear in mind that you may now have to adapt some of your practices, especially those that involve restraints.

Sometimes, BDSM involves playing with pain inflicted by whips, floggers, canes, nipple clamps, or other props. It's not the kind of pain we associate with stubbing your toe. Instead, pain creates extremely intense stimulation, which, when inflicted by someone who knows what he or she is doing, can provide intensely pleasurable sensations.

So what's enjoyable about being spanked? Have you ever had an intense sexual experience and afterward noticed bite marks on your neck of which you had no memory? Your partner bit you hard enough that it bruised you, and all you felt was another jolt of pleasure. If your partner was to bite you that hard outside of a sexual context, it would likely hurt a lot! But when you're sexually aroused, your tolerance for pain soars, and stimulation that you usually feel as pain becomes pleasurable.

BDSM RULES OF ENGAGEMENT

Communicate what you might like to try, and discuss your boundaries *before* your scene.

Establish a "safe" word or signal (such as the "peace" sign) that, when said or shown, immediately stops all activity.

Play sober. You want to be completely aware of what you're doing and not placing your partner in a dangerous or compromising situation.

Be respectful, loving, and caring throughout the scene.

Start slow.

Don't pressure your partner into doing things he or she may not be ready for.

If using restraints, make sure you're not injuring your partner. Check in with your partner along the way to make sure everything is okay.

Always stay clear of the face and lower back (kidneys) when spanking, paddling, or whipping, as you don't want to cause any damage to internal organs or leave any marks on the face that will require an explanation.

Always warm up an area before any flogging, because it lessens the shock to the body; massage works well.

If you're using restraints, only restrain one or two parts. In other words, don't tie his hands, gag his mouth, *and* blindfold him. You have to leave him with a way to communicate.

For more guidelines, visit www.bdsmcircle.com.

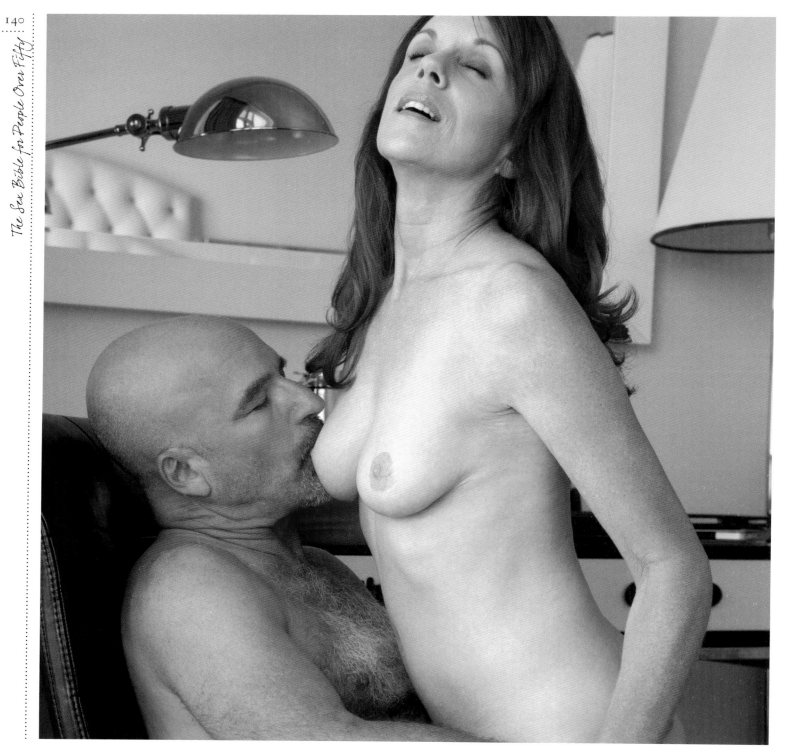

One explanation is that the brain produces endorphins—natural opiates—to compensate for the pain, so that you actually get "high" off the sensation. A good example of this is what athletes experience during periods of high performance. They often describe how they're "hooked on exercise." They, too, enjoy stressing their bodies to get that chemical response.

Proper Use of Props

Props are often part of BDSM play. They can include items you might find around your house, such as ties, ribbons, wooden spoons, or clothespins. Others you can buy—such as floggers, whips, or nipple clamps. Please read up on how to employ any of these objects in BDSM play. If not used carefully and correctly, they can harm you or your partner.

Considerations for the Over-Fifty Kinky Crowd

If you're over fifty, some issues to consider before "playing" include:
• Eyesight: Wear your contact lenses or glasses if you need them. You need to be able to see where you're hitting!
• Hearing loss: You have to be able to hear your partner's safe word if he or she gives

it. Choose a nonverbal signal if you have trouble hearing (or if you're going to gag your partner).
• Joint and muscle flexibility: If you're going to restrain someone, he or she has to be comfortable enough so that the restraints don't inflict pain. Remember that pain only feels good when the person is fully aroused.
• Blood circulation issues: Don't suspend your partner or keep his arms above his head for too long if he has poor blood flow.
• Arthritis: This will make tying proper knots difficult, so choose an activity that you can do with ease.
• Chronic pain: Any activity that aggravates that pain will not be experienced as positive.

Other considerations include:
• Void your bladder before play. As we age, it often becomes more difficult to hold it in, and no one wants to have "an accident" while trying to get out of restraints.
• Don't hold positions for too long. Arms and legs can cramp and get tense.
• Always make sure fragile parts of the body (such as the neck) are supported.
• If you're going to spank or flog, aim for areas that have more cushioning, such as the buttocks.
• Be careful of areas where there is thinning skin, such as the upper arms.

OPEN MARRIAGES

Later in life, some couples decide to experiment with the boundaries of sexual permission. An "open" relationship is a nonmonogamous relationship. It is *not* cheating. Cheating involves betrayal. When a relationship is open, both partners are consenting to the nonmonogamy. They are aware of and okay with extramarital activities. In other words, an open marriage is one that permits sexual relationships outside the normal boundaries of marriage.

Open relationships are about *sex*, not intimacy. This kind of arrangement isn't for everyone. There are many factors to consider before you say, "Yes, let's do this." For example, ask yourself:
• How will I feel if my partner seems to be enjoying his lover more than he enjoys me?
• What if that new partner has more stamina than me, has a bigger penis than me, or is younger than me?
• Can I handle this without jealousy?
• Where are we going to do this—at a hotel, our own home, a swinger's club, or only on vacation?

CASE STUDY: LISA AND TIM

Lisa, forty-nine, and Tim, fifty-three, agreed early on in their marriage that they would stretch their sexual boundaries. They attend mostly public "swingers" parties, meaning that the parties occur in specific nightclubs or bars and are open to the public. These places often have a "private" section where people can have sex with others. Lisa and Tim both agreed that they would not have sex with other people but that they were each allowed to "make out" with whomever they chose. They've never gone further than this, but both say that it's kept the fires burning in their marriage.

RULES FOR NONMONOGAMY

You both decide on the kind of sexual permission to give each other.

You trust each other and don't harbor insecurities that will cause jealousy.

You need to find like-minded new partners who can respect your rules and arrangement.

The needs of the couple outweigh the needs of the one, so if one person is no longer okay with the arrangement, it must stop.

Always practice safe sex with new partners.

Another factor to consider is the other person. When you invite another partner into your "bedroom," you're also inviting in potential personal issues that may complicate your life. Finally, do you publicize to your social network that you're in an open relationship? What about their judgment of you, since monogamy is what our society seems to value, as a rule?

It may take a while to figure out your boundaries and what you're comfortable with. This means that you may make some mistakes, encounter complicated or unexpected situations, and possibly hurt your partner unintentionally. Prepare yourselves for this and remember that forgiveness has to be a part of this arrangement. Open communication is key.

Swinging, the "Lifestyle"
Some couples are part of a community of swingers, or lifestylers, as they now prefer to be called. These couples generally are in long-term, stable relationships and seek out other couples for sexual activity. This practice used to be known as "swapping." One of the most common reasons cited by couples who enter the lifestyle at a later age is to "spice things up" and become adventurous. For most couples this will not be an option, yet those who do engage in it say that their primary relationship is stronger and more exciting than it once was.

Carol and David, both fifty, run a website for lifestylers. A suburban couple with kids (his and hers), and who have been together for six years, they discovered the swinging lifestyle five years ago during a trip to Mexico. They found that it fit so well with how they both wanted to live their sexuality that they decided to make a business out of it (www.venuscouples.com). They enjoy a tremendously active sex life and often organize parties and trips where the focus is on "playing" with other couples. They recently went on a cruise with four thousand other lifestylers.

Says Carol, "This lifestyle works for us because it forces us to talk openly with each other about our sexual needs, desires, and fantasies. We have no secrets. This type of dialogue keeps us on the same page throughout our relationship. And we enjoy letting the other fulfill a sexual fantasy. It's like giving the gift of pleasure. It also makes us feel young. When we dress up sexy and go out on a 'date,' we feel like kids again. We also feel young and sexy when we're at a swingers club and we get to flirt and choose whom we might want to have sex with. We both enjoy the thrill of the chase."

Big Love: *Polyamory*

Polyamory, meaning "multiple loves," is another form of openness. It's a lifestyle that involves the permission to have multiple love relationships. Unlike the "open" relationships described above, these relationships involve more than sex. The premise is that you can love more than one person. In poly relationships, however, there's still generally a primary relationship, but the extramarital activities involve intimate—emotional and sexual—relations with others.

These relationships can be less complicated if you're an older couple, because you're not dealing with trying to explain what you're doing to young children living with you—and you have more free time to invest in multiple relationships.

Couples who live this way often do so because of a strong belief in nonmonogamy, without valuing casual sex. Generally, they are couples who have strong communication skills and who do not experience much jealousy. Couples who choose nonmonogamy later in life tend to do so because they want variety in terms of sex and romantic partners, without the betrayal and secrecy, and ultimately want to stay with their primary partner.

EXPLORING TANTRIC SEX

Tantra is an often misunderstood form of sexuality. The premise behind it is that by removing the focus on orgasm, sex becomes more about connection and intimacy than the desire to fulfill an itch. Movements are slow and deliberate, and there's a focused concentration on breathing. Tantric sex can be the ideal form of sexuality for couples who may have physical issues that get in the way of intimacy.

Sex as a Journey Rather Than a Destination

Some people ask, "If there's no orgasm, what's the point?" Well, when you consider that the average act of penetration lasts a mere five minutes, many people are left with the feeling of "Is that all there is?" after sex.

Tantra means "expansion through awareness" in the Sanskrit language. It's all about the process and journey rather than the orgasm. As a result, the existence or nonexistence of an orgasm is completely unimportant if you regard the whole encounter as a fulfilling, intimate act and not an express lane to climax.

People who are unable to achieve orgasm enjoy Tantra because the pressure to climax is off, and they're able to live in the moment. Tantric sex often lasts for hours because there's no orgasm-oriented goal—although there's no "rule" against having an orgasm.

Tantra Basics

Tantra isn't as simple as it may sound. People commonly study their Tantric techniques over the course of years, learning to master sophisticated breathing techniques, energy flow, and massage.

Typically, the man sits on the bed or in a chair, and his partner sits on top of him. Because the goal is a total body and mind connection, they gaze into each other's eyes. As she lowers herself onto him, he enters her, but there's none of the thrusting we'd normally expect. Gentle rocking movements keep him in a state of erection but not enough to bring him quickly to orgasm.

Some people prefer to breathe in sync with their partner; others inhale when their partner exhales and vice versa. Each partner delicately massages the other's body, stroking from the stomach to the head to keep the energy rising in the body. The kissing is deep and soulful.

You might enjoy putting your right hand over your lover's heart and having him or her do the same to yours. Take the time to breathe slowly and feel the connection between you. Play soft or slow music in the background to accentuate the experience. Light candles or incense if you'd like.

In contrast to regular intercourse, Tantra sex makes it easier to concentrate on the feeling of the penis in the vagina. As with relaxation exercises, where you focus on relaxing every extremity of your body one by one, you'll have a heightened awareness of every tiny movement and sensation. If you're able to climax and you want to, go right ahead. You're the director of your Tantric session.

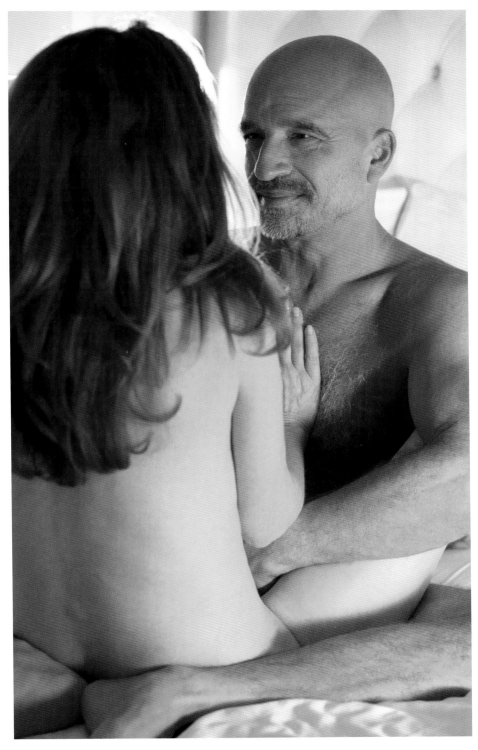

Do I Really Need to Orgasm?

Ask yourself whether an orgasm is becoming less or more important to you. For many people over the age of fifty, orgasm is *not* the sole focus it once was. What we crave is a deeper connection to our partners and to have a more fulfilling love relationship with them. Take a few minutes to reflect on the question of whether or not you could have a fulfilling sex life without orgasm. Could you still be satisfied?

Generally speaking, if you're physically, mentally, and spiritually connected to your loved one, an orgasm is just a bonus to an already very pleasurable experience. If you think about it, when you're focused on the orgasm, you're concentrating more on your own body and pleasure than on your partner's. It's not necessarily a bad thing; it doesn't take anything away from your love for your partner. But by nature, focusing on your own orgasm is a more selfish act than if you have sex without expecting to climax.

In some couples, especially if they've been together for a very long time, sex can become mechanical and completely goal driven. This can be caused by boredom, trouble between the couple, time restraints, or other factors. Tantric sex may just be the tonic that you need to rekindle your love and connection. If you already have a great relationship and sex life, why not consider adding Tantra from time to time to experience a different dimension?

Tantric Checklist

• Take 10 minutes a day to connect and communicate with your partner.
• Slow things down.
• Keep your eyes open and gaze at each other while you practice deep breathing.

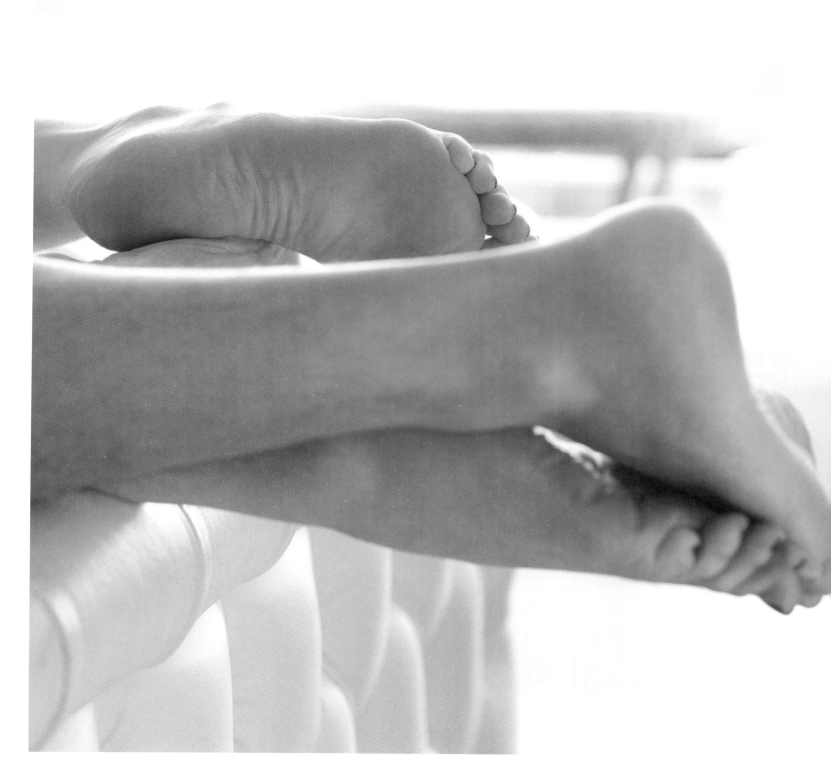

10 ♂♀ *Great Sex Is Just the Beginning*

It's often said that sex is complicated, and to some extent, that could be considered accurate. Sexual experiences are wrought with challenges right from the start. Children begin discovering their genitals only to be told by parents and teachers that they shouldn't touch themselves. By the time we hit puberty, hormones are raging but we lack the maturity and social finesse to harness them. When we have our first sexual experiences, they're often accompanied by shyness, insecurities, body image issues, and a range of complicated emotions.

"My husband loved *Fifty Shades of Grey*! He didn't read it, mind you, but he reaped all the benefits of me reading it!"

"I thought that when my kids all moved out, my life would be very lonely. Now my husband and I are having a rekindled romance!"

In our twenties, we're supposedly at our sexual peak. Some people use that time to gain as much experience as possible with as many partners as possible. Others are already actively working on pairing up with the goal of a lifelong commitment. The majority of couples begin having children at some point in their twenties or early thirties. And with those children comes great responsibility. Free time, privacy, and energy are at a premium, quite often diminishing the opportunity or even desire for sex. The last time I checked, the age of majority was eighteen, so that's a lot of years to sacrifice your sex life.

By the time the kids move out of the house, couples are already in what we consider middle age. Many people find themselves feeling like they did when they were teenagers—insecure and suffering from body image issues. We've put on a few pounds, hair is growing in the strangest of places, the C-section or other surgery scar is still visible, and we realize that we're far from being physically perfect.

But you now have the maturity to understand that none of these realities is that important. Your boobs hang lower than they ever did? Big deal. You have stretch marks on your belly? Evidence of experience. Those few extra pounds? More to love.

That's the beauty of being over fifty. You've gained enough experience and knowledge over your life span to understand that more often than not, sex is an expression of feelings that supersedes any bodily changes. Your partner turns you on with his mind more than he does with his body. You can enjoy yourself and have fun without the pressure.

Unfortunately, saying no to sex can become a bad habit. You can always find excuses not to have sex. Well, no more excuses, no more neglecting your relationship and your sexual selves. If you've read this book, then you're clearly ready and willing, and now you have some tools to use. Remember that we're in control of our sex lives, and we can have it for as long as we choose to.

> "I'm more in love with my husband now than I was twenty-five years ago, and the sex is awesome!"

WHEN TO SEEK HELP

Sometimes you have the desire and the willingness to be sexual, but there's a hurdle that you can't seem to overcome. That's where professionals such as sex therapists come in. The earlier you seek help and advice on the issue of sex, the more time you will have to spend on a fulfilling sex life.

WHEN TO SEEK SEX/ COUPLES THERAPY

• If you're experiencing serious relationship difficulties that you're unable to resolve.
• If the subject of sex often comes up but you make no progress.
• If either of you has unresolved issues that are affecting your relationship.
• If your sexual relationship has never been satisfactory.
• If you experience any sexual difficulties for a long period of time.
• If you routinely avoid sex.

Over the course of the past twenty-three years, I've had the privilege of helping many couples. It's always so gratifying to watch the growth or rebirth of a relationship. I've seen women discover their sexuality for the first time—or rediscover it after a difficult spell. I've heard from older couples that they never would have thought that sex could get so much better with age. I've seen the wonderment in the eyes of clients who have discovered a new sexual activity.

I often tell my clients, "You're here in my office because of your strength, not your weakness." It takes strength to admit that we need help. It takes strength to open your mind and your heart to a different way of doing things. I've also witnessed, time and again, that when there's a will, there's always a way.

In every other area of life, people know that their goals and dreams take persistence and preparation. However, when it comes to their love lives and sex lives, there is a comforting belief system that it will somehow all work out. Well, there are times when it doesn't all work out and you need to take some action, show a little initiative, and follow some solid sex advice. The great news is that you have already taken the first step by reading this book and making something wonderful happen for you and your partner.

It's true that relationships take work. But that work keeps the relationship alive, much like a plant requires nurturing and care to blossom. I urge you to put the time and energy into taking the knowledge you've gleaned from this book and investing it in your relationship. Bear in mind that although age is quantifiably measurable, great sex is timeless.

With any luck, you'll find yourself like this client: "I'm having the best sex of my life! I feel like at fifty, I finally have my life and body back. It's time for me now!"

REFERENCES

CHAPTER 2

Block, J. *Sex Over 50*. Mira Loma, CA: Parker Publishing, 1999.

Burleson, M.H., Trevathan, W.R., and Todd, M. "In the mood for love or vice versa? Exploring the relations among sexual activity, physical affection, affect, and stress in the daily lives of mid-aged women." *Archives of Sexual Behavior* 36, no. 3 (June 2007): 357–68.

CHAPTER 3

Astbury-Ward, E. M. "Menopause, sexuality and culture: Is there a universal experience?" *Sexual and Relationship Therapy* 18, no. 4 (2003): 437–45.

Birnbaum, G. E., Cohen, O, and Wertheimer, V. "Is it all about intimacy? Age, menopausal status, and women's sexuality." *Personal Relationships* 14, no. 1 (April 2007): 167–85.

Dabrowska, J, Drosdzol, A, Skrzypulec, V, and Plinta, R. "Physical activity and sexuality in perimenopausal women." *The European Journal of Contraception and Reproductive Health Care* 15, no. 6 (December 2010): 423–32.

Domoney, C, Currie, H, Panay, N, Maamari, R, and Nappi, R.E. "The CLOSER Survey: Impact of postmenopausal vaginal discomfort on women and male partners in the UK." *Menopause International* 19, no. 2 (June 2013): 69–76.

Kegel, A.H. "Sexual Functions of the Pubococcygeus Muscle," *Western Journal of Surgery, Obstetrics & Gynecology* 60 (1952): 521–24.

Kolod, S. "Menopause and sexuality." *Contemporary Psychoanalysis* 45, no. 1 (2009): 26–43.

Canadian Institute for Laser Surgery, www.lasermontreal.com.

Millheiser, L.S., Pauls, R.N., Herbst, S.J., and Chen, B.H. "Radiofrequency treatment of vaginal laxity after vaginal delivery: Nonsurgical vaginal tightening." *Journal of Sexual Medicine* 7, no. 9 (September 2010): 3088–95.

Pauls, R.N., Fellner, A.N., and Davila, G.W. "Vaginal laxity: A poorly understood quality of life problem; a survey of physician members of the International Urogynecological Association." *International Urogynecology Journal* 23, no. 10 (October 2012): 1435–48.

Simon, J.A., Nappi, R.E., Kingsberg, S.A., Maamari, R, and Brown, V. "Clarifying vaginal atrophy's impact on sex and relationships (CLOSER) survey: Emotional and physical impact of vaginal discomfort on North American post-menopausal women and their partners." *Menopause* (February 2014): 21(2); 137–142.

Society of Obstetricians and Gynaecologists of Canada. "SOGC clinical practice guidelines. The detection and management of vaginal atrophy. Number 145, May 2004." *International Journal of Gynecology & Obstetrics* 88, no. 2 (February 2005): 222–8.

CHAPTER 4

Abstract presented at the American Urological Association (AUA) 2012 Annual Scientific Meeting: Abstract 1486. Presented May 22, 2012, San Diego.

Carrier, S. "Canadian sexual satisfaction survey 2003." *Journal of Sexual & Reproductive Medicine* 3, suppl. B (Winter 2003).

Center for Male Reproductive Medicine and Microsurgery, Cornell University, www.cornellurology.com/about/treatment-centers/center-for-male-reproductive-medicine-microsurgery.

CNN. "Erectile dysfunction: The leading indicator of heart disease in men," http://thechart.blogs.cnn.com/2011/08/17/erectile-dysfunction-the-leading-indicator-of-heart-disease-in-men.

Department of Urology, Weill Cornell Medical College. "Vacuum Devices for Erectile Dysfunction," www.cornellurology.com/clinical-conditions/erectile-dysfunction/vacuum-devices.

Friedman, D.M. *A Mind of Its Own: A Cultural History of the Penis.* New York: The Free Press, 2001.

IMS Brogan, Canadian CompuScript. MAT December 2013.

Kim, S. C., Chang, I. H., and Jeon, H. J. (2003). "Preference for oral sildenafil or intracavernosal injection in patients with erectile dysfunction already using intracavernosal injection for > 1 year." *BJU International*, 92(3), 277–280.

Levine, L.A., Estrada, C. R., and Morgentaler, A. (2001). "Mechanical reliability and safety of, and patient satisfaction with the Ambicor inflatable penile prosthesis: results of a 2 center study." *The Journal of Urology*, 166(3), 932–937.

McCarthy, B, and McCarthy, E. *Rekindling Desire: A Step-by-Step Program to Help Low-Sex and No-Sex Marriages.* London: Routledge, 2003.

McCullough, A.R., Barada, J.H. , Fawzy, A, Guay, A.T., and Hatzichristou, D. "Achieving treatment optimization with sildenafil citrate (Viagra) in patients with erectile dysfunction." *Urology* 60, suppl. 2 (September 2002): 28–38.

Tal, R, Jacks, L.M., Elkin, E, Mulhall, J.P. "Penile implant utilization following treatment for prostate cancer: analysis of the SEER-Medicare database." *Journal of Sexual Medecine*, 2011, June:8(6): 1797–804.

MedicineNet, www.medicinenet.com.

Michael A. Werner, M.D., F.A.C.S., urologist and specialist in sexual dysfuntion, www.wernermd.com.

CHAPTER 5
Arackal, B.S., and Benegal, V. "Prevalence of sexual dysfunction in male subjects with alcohol dependence." *Indian Journal of Psychiatry* 49, no. 2 (April–June 2007): 109–12.

Basson, R. "A model of women's sexual arousal." *Journal of Sex & Marital Therapy* 28, no. 1 (January–February 2002): 1–10.

DeLamater, J, and Moorman, S.M. "Sexual behavior in later life." *Journal of Aging and Health* 19 (December 2007): 921–45.

Goldstein, A, and Brandon, M. *Reclaiming Desire: 4 Keys to Finding Your Lost Libido.* Emmaus, PA: Rodale: 2004.

Kalra, G, Subramanyam, A, and Pinto, C. "Sexuality: Desire, activity and intimacy in the elderly." *Indian Journal of Psychiatry* 53, no. 4 (October–December 2011): 300–306.

Krychman, M. *100 Questions & Answers about Women's Sexual Wellness and Vitality.* Sudbury, MA: Jones & Bartlett Learning, 2010.

Levine, S. B. "The nature of sexual desire: A clinician's perspective." *Archives of Sexual Behavior* 32, no. 3 (2003): 279–85.

Pat Love and Associates, www.PatLove.com.

Perel, E. *Mating in Captivity.* New York: Harper Perennial, 2007.

Starr, B.D., and Bakur Weiner, M. *The Starr-Weiner Report on Sex and Sexuality in the Mature Years.* New York: Mcgraw-Hill, 1982.

Trompeter, S.E., Bettencourt, R, and Barrett-Connor, E. "Sexual activity and satisfaction in healthy community-dwelling older women." *American Journal of Medicine* 125, no. 1 (January 2012): 37–43.

CHAPTER 6
Grufferman, B.H. "The Best of Everything After 50," www.FrankTalks.com.

CHAPTER 7
Krychman, M.L. *100 Questions & Answers about Women's Sexual Wellness and Vitality.* Sudbury, MA: Jones & Bartlett Learning, 2010.

The University of Chicago Medicine website, www.uchospitals.edu/online-library/content=CDR62862.

CHAPTER 8
Dan Waldston, massage therapist, Montreal, www.therapeutic-massage.ca.

McBride, K.R., and Fortenberry, J.D. "Heterosexual Anal Sexuality and Anal Sex Behaviors: A Review." *Journal of Sex Research,* 47, no. 2 (2010): 123–36.

Morin, J. *Anal Pleasure & Health.* San Francisco, CA: Down There Press, 1998.

Das, A. "Masturbation in the United States." *Journal of Sex & Marital Therapy,* 33 (2007): 301–317).

Herbenick, D, et al. "Sexual Behavior in the United Sates: Results from a national probability sample of men and women ages 14–94." *Journal of Sexual Medicine* 2010; 7 (suppl 5): 255–65.

CHAPTER 9
The BDSM Circle, www.bdsmcircle.com.

The Fantasy Box, www.thefantasybox.com.

Kuriansky, J. *The Complete Idiot's Guide to Tantric Sex.* 2nd ed. New York: Penguin Group, 2004.

Venus Couples, www.venuscouples.com.

ACKNOWLEDGMENTS

There are so many people that I am grateful for in my life and who have contributed to who I am today. First, I would like to thank Jill Alexander of Quarto, who took a chance on me and was always right behind me to get the book done. In the writing of this book I had two wonderful guides, both authors in their own right: Cynthia Badiey, who helped me organize the content, and my good friend and colleague Frank Kermit, who gave me so much encouragement and guidance throughout the process.

There are several people I consider my primary mentors, who have been with me since the beginning of my career. Dr. Pierre Assalian, who trained me in sex therapy and took me under his wing, and helped me soar in the field. I am eternally indebted to him for his love and support. To Pat Rubin, whose approach I love and who inspired me and taught me how to work with couples, thank you.

Thanks to Rick Moffat, my radio mentor, who put me on the airwaves when I was a young twenty-something fresh-out-of-school therapist and who is still my biggest fan. To my CJAD/Passion listeners and to my clients, you taught me so much about humility and compassion. I owe the career I so love to all of you. Thank you for making me a part of your lives for so many years.

My gratitude goes to my assistants/interns, Genevieve LaRoche, Malissa Veroni, and Tanya D'Amours, who devoted precious hours of their time to helping me.

To my wonderful colleagues of many years who are also my friends and whose support, supervision, and listening skills have meant the world to me: Sharon Brodie, Stephanie Mitelman, Cleve Zeigler, Rebecca Puterman, Pascale Brillon, Marc Lemieux, Marilyn Wilchesky, Hélène Côte, Steve Solomon, Kevin Hayes, Stéphane Bensoussan, Marc Ravart, Jack Strulovitch, Serge Carrier, Clifford Albert, Dan Delmar, Gilles Ouimet, Patty Terrone, Frank Mondeosé, Teresa Norris, Kelly Borbridge, and Linda Shore.

I must mention the professors who taught me so much, and who inspired me to continue in the field of psychology and sexology: Jean Côte, Paulos Milkias, Carol Christensen, Sydney Duder, Gail Wyatt, and Ellen Moss.

I have a network of incredible friends, couples, and "sisters" (the majority over fifty) with whom I've spent countless hours discussing sex and relationships. I learned from them, too, the struggles of married life, their fears, and for many, the great sex they were having. They told me what they needed to see in a book about sex that was designed for them.

And finally, how do you go about thanking family? Thank you is just not enough.

To my siblings, who know how to stick together: The pride and love we feel for each other is a true gift.

To my parents: No words can express the depth of gratitude I feel for their undying support during every step I took. Even when I shocked them with my choice of career in the "sex field," they got over it and beamed with pride. Although my father found it too difficult to listen to his little girl on the radio talking about anal or oral sex (and way beyond), my mom has been a nightly listener for fourteen years, and my biggest fan.

To my husband, my rock: Without his nurturance and the ease with which he handled our household when I worked late, I would never have been able to accomplish what I set out to do. He has always been proud to let me shine. His patience, and his ability to "get me" and let me be me, has been a wonderful source of empowerment.

To my girls, my pride and joy: You are my greatest accomplishment. I feel so privileged to have birthed and mothered you. Watching you grow is a daily inspiration.

ABOUT THE AUTHOR

Laurie Betito, Ph.D., known as "Dr. Laurie,"
is a clinical psychologist with a specialty
in sex therapy, and has been a practicing
psychotherapist for the past twenty-five
years. For the past twenty-three years she has
been dispensing sex and relationship advice
on radio and television programs. She is a
regular contributor to various magazines,
newspapers, and television shows. She
is heard nightly in Montreal on CJAD
800AM (www.cjad.com, to listen live);
her show "Passion" has been on the air for
fifteen years.

Dr. Laurie is also president of the Sexual
Health Network of Quebec (formerly
Planned Parenthood), and past president of
the Canadian Sex Research Forum.

INDEX